An Atlas of
SURGICAL APPROACHES
to the BONES
of the DOG and CAT

D. L. Piermattei, D.V.M., M.S.

Associate Professor of Veterinary Medicine and Surgery
College of Veterinary Medicine, Texas A. & M. University

R. G. Greeley, D.V.M., M.S.

Associate Professor of Veterinary Anatomy
College of Veterinary Medicine, Texas A. & M. University

W. B. SAUNDERS COMPANY   *Philadelphia and London,*

W. B. Saunders Company: West Washington Square
                          Philadelphia, Pa.   19105

                          12 Dyott Street
                          London, WC1A   1DB

                          833 Oxford Street
                          Toronto, Ontario M8Z 5T9, Canada

Listed here is the latest translated edition of this book together with the language of the transla-
tion and the publisher.

French (1st Edition) — La Maloine,
              Paris, France

An Atlas of Surgical Approaches to the Bones of the Dog and Cat   ISBN 0-7216-7240-X

Print No.:   12   11   10   9

Dedicated to those veterinary surgeons
who pioneered the anatomic approach to surgery
and made this volume possible

PREFACE

Anatomical study has one application for the man of science who loves knowledge for its own sake, another for him who values it only to demonstrate that nature does nought in vain, a third for one who provides himself from anatomy with data for investigating a function, physical or mental, and yet another for the practitioner who has to remove splinters and missiles efficiently.

GALEN

In the course of several years' experience in teaching small animal surgery to veterinary students, a need for well illustrated material on the surgical anatomy of the skeletal system became very apparent. Until now, this material has only been available in scattered articles and portions of books, and even there the quality of photography and artwork has often been a limiting factor in the lucidity of the instructions. Investigators reporting orthopedic problems in the veterinary literature have tended to devote a great deal of attention to the pathology and repair of the lesion, while dismissing the problem of anatomic exposure of the area with a cursory explanation and perhaps a single line drawing. The truth is that an adequate, atraumatic, and anatomically sound exposure of the affected bone or bones is at least 50 per cent of the battle in most orthopedic procedures. It is our hope, therefore, that this book will fill a void in the student's and the practitioner's bookshelves and allow them to have available in one place directions for approaches to all the bones.

The particular exposures chosen for inclusion here do not represent every possible method of approaching a given area. Rather, they represent methods that have proven useful in the clinical practice of the senior author. Multiple techniques are presented for certain areas, and some approaches overlap others in terms of the region of bone exposed. The surgeon must therefore use his judgment in choosing an approach, selecting the one most readily applicable to the problem at hand. When multiple techniques are available, the surgeon should try each of them and select the one with which he is most comfortable.

No attempt has been made to use proper names for the procedures or to accredit individuals as original investigators. It is extremely difficult to assign priority for the original description to a number of these procedures, and many have derived from techniques used in man. In the same vein, no claim for originality is made by us for having developed any of these operations. An anatomically descriptive title has been used for each approach in an attempt to clearly identify the utility of a particular procedure.

All artwork in this book has been done by Dr. Greeley. The drawings are original and were produced from dissections performed on cadavers. As each dissection progressed, rough sketches were compiled and photographs were made. A description of each procedure was dictated as dissections were accomplished, and these descriptions became the basis for the text accompanying the drawings. Finished drawings were made from the rough sketches and the photographs. Anatomic detail was reproduced in the final drawing as faithfully as clarity would permit. *Anatomy of the Dog* by Miller, Christensen, and Evans (W. B. Saunders Co., 1964) was used as a guide for nomenclature and identification of structures. Wherever possible, anglicized names were used in preference to Latin terms, as it was felt that they are in more common use by veterinary surgeons. Dissections were repeated on cats and, where appropriate, variations from the dog were noted in both text and drawings.

As always, much credit must go to those who, by various means, have assisted with the production of this book. We are most grateful to our wives and families for their forbearance, as most of the work was done evenings and weekends. The facilities of the Department of Veterinary Medicine and Surgery, Texas A. & M. University, were made available through the cooperation of Dr. M. R. Calliham. The aid and encouragement of Dr. John H. Milliff proved invaluable. The manuscript was typed cheerfully and ably by Mrs. Ellen Hux. Every procedure was reviewed and criticized by Dr. Leonard Hurov, who also supplied the procedure for the "Approach to the Distal End of the Radius and the Radiocarpal Joint." From Dr. Greeley there is a special expression of thanks to Mr. William Osburn, Medical Art Director, W. B. Saunders Co., without whose advice and help this book might never have materialized. Lastly, Dr. Piermattei wishes to express his debt for the surgical training and inspiration supplied by Dr. Wade O. Brinker.

D. L. P.

R. G. G.

College Station, Texas

CONTENTS

SECTION I

SECTION II

SECTION III

Page vii

SECTION IV

SECTION V

I | GENERAL CONSIDERATIONS

ATTRIBUTES OF AN ACCEPTABLE APPROACH TO A BONE OR JOINT

The bones and joints must be exposed in a manner that insures the preservation of the anatomic and physiologic functions of the area invaded. Major blood vessels, nerves, and tendons must be avoided or protected. Maximal use must be made of muscle separation with incision of muscles being avoided whenever possible. Transection of muscle bellies must be kept at an absolute minimum; tenotomy of the muscles at their origin or insertion is much preferred. Skin incisions must be made in such a manner that the vascular supply to the incisions is not impaired. No pedicles or sharp angles should exist in the incision since these points commonly undergo avascular necrosis and produce excessive scar formation. A cosmetically acceptable scar should be the goal when operating on pet animals. In general, the procedure should not add unnecessary trauma to that which the injured area has already sustained.

FACTORS TO CONSIDER WHEN CHOOSING AN APPROACH

THE AREA TO BE EXPOSED

The problem of choosing the best approach is easily solved in some instances. For example, there is only one logical way to expose the midshaft of the femur (see the Approach to the Shaft of the Femur, p. 104), and therefore the decision is easily made. Other areas do not lend themselves to such clear-cut answers. In some instances, the choice is purely a matter of the surgeon's personal preference. The area of the hip joint perhaps illustrates this best, there being many choices for exposure of this general area. Ultimately it rests with the surgeon to try all approaches and to adapt the ones best suited to him.

BREED, SIZE, AND CONFORMATION OF THE ANIMAL

The area of the hip may also be used to illustrate the relationship of the animal's physique to the problem. We are speaking here not only of the size but also of the body type and the degree of obesity of the patient. As an example, the Approach to the Hip Joint Through a Craniolateral Incision (p. 86) serves very nicely as an approach for femoral head ostectomy in the small breeds and in lean animals up to approximately 30 pounds in body weight. However, in the large breeds or in obese animals of the smaller breeds, this procedure affords only limited exposure owing to either the massiveness of the musculature or the thickness of gluteal fat.

THE TYPE OF FRACTURE OR LUXATION

Multiple injuries will require multiple approaches or perhaps a combination of methods. By scanning the approaches to various areas of a bone, one can easily note those which lend themselves to combining. An example might be a combination of one of the procedures for the hip or pelvis with the Approach to the Shaft of the Femur.

ASSOCIATED SOFT-TISSUE DAMAGE OR INFECTION

When a choice of approaches exists, the extent and location of associated injuries can influence the choice of approach. An attempt is always made to avoid exposing bone through an existing skin wound or sinus tract. The purpose of this is to prevent the transfer of infected or infective material to the bone and the surrounding deep structures. The same reasoning is applied to open (compound) fractures. The temptation to extend the original wound in the skin and muscle to expose the bone must be overcome.

ASEPTIC TECHNIQUE

The keystone upon which success or failure of open bone and joint surgery rests is meticulous devotion to the ritual of *aseptic technique*. True enough, gentle handling of tissues and an anatomically sound approach are of utmost importance, but they go for nought in the presence of wound infection or osteomyelitis. The incidence of these sequelae can be reduced to almost zero by a combination of rigid asepsis and the use of antibiotics pre- and postoperatively.

A detailed discussion of the methods of sterilization is beyond the scope of this book. In general, autoclaving at 250° F. and 15 lb. pressure and with a contact time of 12 to 15 minutes is the most practical way of sterilizing instruments and cloth materials such as drapes and gowns. Sterilizer indicators which undergo a color change when exposed to proper sterilization conditions should be used in *every* autoclave load. This indicator should be placed inside the largest pack to insure that such sterilization conditions are reached. Total time in the autoclave is different from contact time; total time is that which is sufficient for steam penetration of the largest pack for the minimum contact time of 12 to 15 minutes. Sterilizer indicators are the only means of establishing the correct total time.

When the sterile instruments, drapes, and gowns are available, the animal must be properly prepared and positioned and then adequately draped to prevent contamination of the surgical field. The reader is referred to the discussion of these techniques by Archibald et al.* and Leonard.†

SURGICAL PRINCIPLES

If it is assumed that aseptic technique is scrupulously practiced, the success or

*Archibald, J., *et al.*: Canine Surgery. 1st Archibald Ed., Santa Barbara, American Veterinary Publications, Inc., 1965.
†Leonard, E. P.: Orthopedic Surgery of the Dog and Cat. Philadelphia, W. B. Saunders Co., 1960.

failure of an open approach devolves to the surgeon's skill in handling tissues *atraumatically*. Although many of the methods herein described are well known to the experienced surgeon, it is hoped that this review will be useful to him in addition to serving as an introduction to this subject for the student.

INCISING AND RETRACTING SKIN AND SUBCUTANEOUS TISSUES

The skin and subcutaneous fascia are incised cleanly and completely before an attempt is made to pick up bleeding vessels. The incision will gape widely when all the subcutaneous fascia is cut, and subsequent eversion of the cut edges facilitates the clamping of bleeders. Meticulous hemostasis is necessary for optimal skin healing.

In most cases subcutaneous fat is incised on the same line as is the skin. The fat is separated down to the deep fascial layer which lies directly on the muscles. It is usually necessary to bluntly separate fat from fascia by the undermining technique shown in Figure 1. This method allows the skin to be widely retracted with minimal interference with its blood supply and exposes the fascia to allow the visualization necessary for the proposed fascial incision.

Hemostatic (crushing) clamps should never be applied to the cut edges of the skin and even Allis forceps are best fastened to subcutaneous fascia to avoid possible trauma. The use of retractors is highly encouraged as a means of avoiding tissue damage. The most useful of these are shown in Figure 2. The Gelpi self-retaining retractor is virtually a third hand for the surgeon working alone.

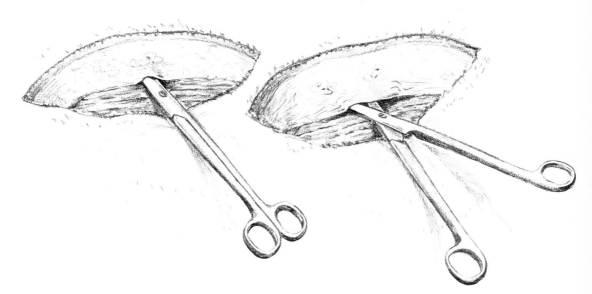

FIGURE 1. Undermining skin and subcutaneous fascia and fat by using Mayo scissors and blunt dissection technique.

INCISING AND RETRACTING DEEP FASCIA

Deep fascia may be loosely adherent to the musculature and may actually slide freely over the muscles, as with the fascia lata, or it may be tightly adherent to the deep structures and difficult to separate from the muscle sheaths. The latter condition is particularly true distal to the elbow and the stifle joint.

The method of incising movable fascia to avoid damaging deep structures is depicted in Figure 3. Tightly adherent fascia is incised with the scalpel, with care being taken to make the incisions directly over muscle separations whenever possible. (See Approach to the Proximal Shaft of the Radius, p. 64.) Fascia is rarely retracted by itself, but rather it is usually retracted with the muscles exposed by the fascial incision.

MUSCLE SEPARATION, ELEVATION, AND RETRACTION

Muscles are separated and elevated from the bone in order to obtain exposure of the bone. The incision of muscles is avoided wherever possible, and tenotomy is held to a minimum. Nothing contributes more to an early return of function than intelligent and gentle handling of muscles.

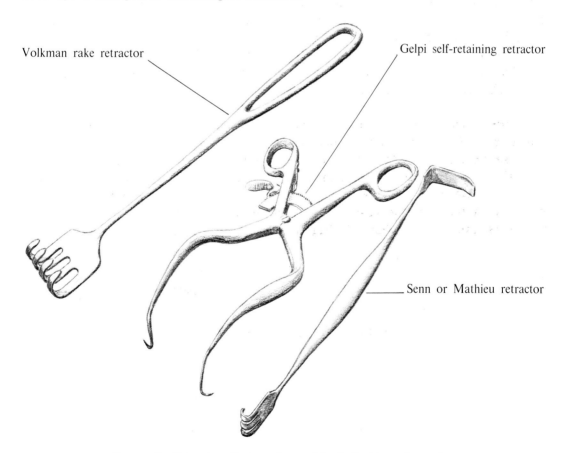

Volkman rake retractor

Gelpi self-retaining retractor

Senn or Mathieu retractor

FIGURE 2. Retractors that can be used for both skin and muscle.

Page 5

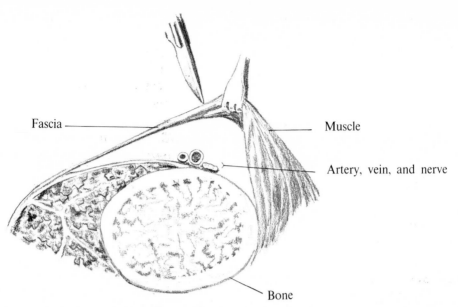

Fascia ——————————————— Muscle

Artery, vein, and nerve

Bone

FIGURE 3. Method of incising deep fascia. The muscle sheath is grasped with forceps and lifted to elevate the fascia from deeper structures.

Muscles are held against the bone by the deep fascia that surrounds the trunk and limbs like a tube. When this fascia is incised, muscles are relatively free except at their origins and insertions. The space between muscles is occupied by rather loose fascial tissue called the intermuscular septum. Bellies of adjacent muscles rarely adhere to one another. Therefore, to separate muscles after the incision of the deep fascia, it is necessary to divide only the intermuscular septa. This is accomplished as shown in Figure 4.

Once the muscles have been separated from one another they must be elevated and retracted. In some cases muscles are easily elevated from underlying bone because there are no extensive periosteal attachments in the area. As an example, the bellies of the vastus lateralis and vastus intermedius muscles are easily separated from the shaft of the femur (see Approach to the Shaft of the Femur, p. 104) by bluntly separating the loose periosteal attachments of the muscular fascia in a manner similar to that shown in Figure 4.

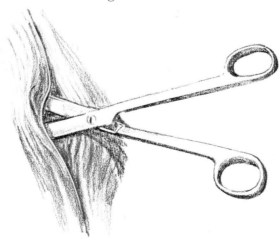

FIGURE 4. Blunt dissection of an intermuscular septum.

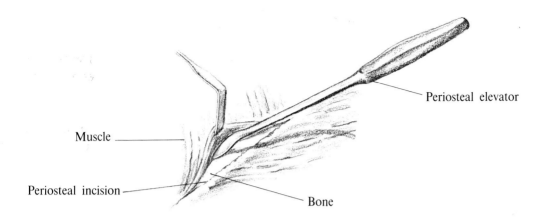

Muscle

Periosteal incision

Bone

Periosteal elevator

FIGURE 5. Subperiosteal elevation of a muscle.

In areas where the muscle is more firmly adherent to the bone it must be elevated in a different manner. Subperiosteal elevation allows muscle to be freed from bone at its origin or insertion without disturbing the muscle fibers. The periosteum is incised and undermined with a periosteal elevator or with the rounded end of the scalpel handle (Fig. 5). Since the periosteum of the dog is rather thin and firmly attached in the area of muscular attachments, its elevation is difficult.

Another form of muscular attachment to bone is the fleshy attachment, in which muscular fascia is attached to the periosteum over a large area as is well illustrated by the origin of the middle gluteal muscle on the iliac crest. Fleshy attachments are elevated by the incision of the fascial connection with the periosteum. The scalpel blade or bone chisel is held almost flat against the bone and the muscle is separated with a "shaving" action.

Finally, in some cases muscles are freed by incising their tendon or aponeurosis of origin or insertion on the bone. This technique is called tenotomy. In most cases sufficient stump is left attached to the bone so that sutures can be placed to re-unite the tendon (see illustration E of Plate 13, Approach to the Shoulder Joint and Distal End of the Scapula, p. 41). In other cases the tendon or aponeurosis is severed close to the bone and no attempt is made at suturing. The best example of this is the elevation of the lumbar muscles from the lumbar vertebrae in the Approach to the Thoracolumbar Vertebrae and Intervertebral Discs Through a Dorsal Incision (p. 26).

After the muscles have been elevated they are retracted and held with muscle retractors. The retractors shown in Figure 2 are quite adequate although there are many other types available. At least one self-retaining and one hand-held retractor are necessary for adequate exposure. A person operating without an assistant could well use two self-retaining retractors.

In the course of separating and elevating muscles, many large blood vessels and major nerve trunks will be encountered in the fascial planes between muscles. These structures must obviously be preserved at all cost.

Whenever possible the nerve or vessel is retracted with an adjoining muscle; this technique takes advantage of the muscle as padding and also prevents undue stretching of the vessel. On occasion these structures must be retracted by themselves in order to achieve adequate exposure of underlying structures. In such a case the vessel or nerve is carefully freed from its enveloping fascia by blunt dissection. A mosquito hemostat is very useful for this dissection since its use avoids the accidental severing of structures which is possible with dissection scissors. When the vessel or nerve has been sufficiently loosened, 1/4-inch umbilical tape is passed around the structure and is then used to maintain traction. This practice is considerably less traumatic than retraction with a metal instrument.

CLOSURE

Joint Capsule. This tissue supports sutures well. Interrupted stitches are always used because of their reliability and safety. If nonabsorbable material is used, care should be taken to prevent suture material from penetrating the synovial membrane and thus entering the joint space. This situation can produce considerable damage to joint cartilage if the suture material contacts the cartilage because of movement of the joint. The stitch is placed so that the needle penetrates only the outer fibrous layer of the joint capsule and emerges on the cut surface between the fibrous and synovial layers. Alternatively, a Lembert pattern may be used, again with the needle penetrating only the fibrous layers.

Muscles. Sutures tend to cut and pull through this relatively soft tissue. A horizontal mattress pattern (Fig. 6) offers the best resistance against being pulled out should it be necessary to suture fleshy portions of muscles. The external fascial

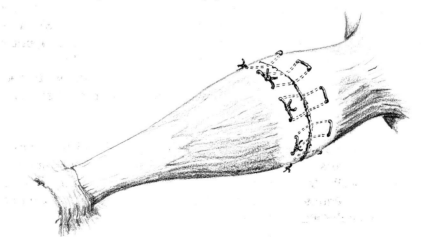

FIGURE 6. Horizontal mattress pattern used to appose a transected muscle. The sutures are placed in external fascia around the muscle belly.

Page 8

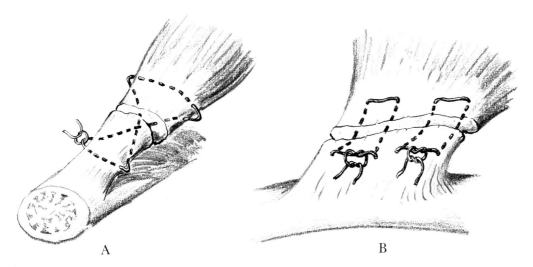

A   B

FIGURE 7. *A*, Bunnell pattern used in a round tendon. *B*, Horizontal mattress pattern used in a flattened tendon or aponeurosis.

sheath of the muscle is the strongest part of muscle tissue and thus is most important in supporting sutures.

Tendons. Although tendons are dense and strong because of the longitudinal and parallel arrangement of their fibers, most stitches tend to cut through them. The classic Bunnell pattern is used in a round tendon (Fig 7*a*) and the horizontal mattress pattern in a flattened tendon or aponeurosis (Fig. 7*b*).

Deep Fascia. No special precautions need be taken here as this tissue holds sutures well. Simple interrupted or simple running patterns work equally well,

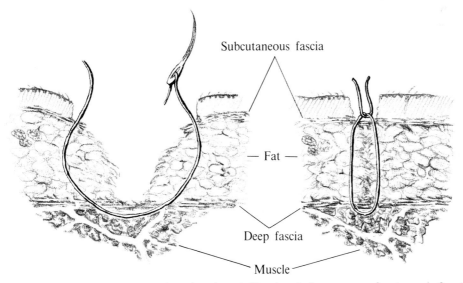

Subcutaneous fascia

— Fat —

Deep fascia

Muscle

FIGURE 8. Method of placing sutures in subcutis. *A*, Simple stitch engages subcutaneous fascia, fat, and muscular or deep fascia. *B*, When stitch is pulled tight it apposes all subcutaneous tissues and eliminates dead space and thereby prevents the formation of serum pockets.

Page 9

although the continuous pattern does not have the safety factor of interrupted stitches.

Subcutaneous Fascia and Fat. Proper closure of this layer is important for two reasons: (1) the space created by incising and undermining the fat fills with serum unless the space is obliterated and (2) closure of the fascia can relieve most of the tension on skin sutures. Simple interrupted or continuous patterns are used. The method of placing the suture is illustrated in Figure 8.

Skin. Simple interrupted sutures are the usual choice in the closure of skin, although many prefer one of the mattress patterns – either horizontal or vertical. Interrupted stitches are the rule in skin closure.

II | THE HEAD

APPROACH TO THE BODY OF THE MANDIBLE

INDICATION:

Open reduction of comminuted fractures of the mandible.

DESCRIPTION OF PROCEDURE:

A. The skin incision is made slightly lateral to the ventral midline of the mandible from the level of the canine tooth to the level of the molar teeth.

The flat and very thin platysma muscle will be incised with the subcutaneous fascia and is then retracted with the fascia and skin.

B. Dorsal retraction of the platysma and skin exposes the body of the mandible.

CLOSURE:

The platysma and subcutaneous fascia are closed in one layer.

PLATE 1. APPROACH TO THE BODY OF THE MANDIBLE

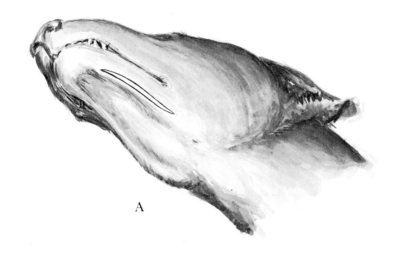

A

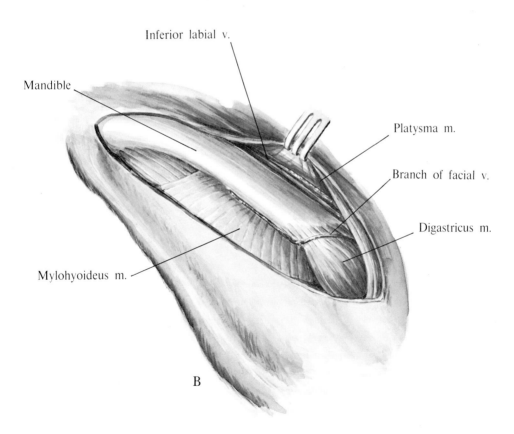

Inferior labial v.

Mandible

Platysma m.

Branch of facial v.

Digastricus m.

Mylohyoideus m.

B

APPROACH TO THE DORSOLATERAL SURFACE
OF THE SKULL

INDICATIONS:

   1. Open reduction of fractures of the frontal and parietal bones and the dorsal parts of the sphenoid and temporal bones.

   2. Exposure of cerebral hemispheres.

DESCRIPTION OF PROCEDURE:

A. The midline skin incision extends from the external occipital protuberance to the level of the eyes. As the subcutaneous fascia is incised and retracted, three muscles are immediately encountered. Rostrally these are the frontalis and interscutularis, the fibers of which run transversely, and caudally the occipitalis with its fibers running parallel to the midline.

B. These muscles are incised on the midline and retracted with the skin. The temporalis muscle is covered by a layer of dense fascia, which is incised on the lateral side of the sagittal and frontal crests. The incision is then deepened to include the periosteum. One or both sides are incised depending on the type of exposure desired.

C. The temporalis is elevated from the skull subperiosteally and retracted laterally.

D. For bilateral exposure, both muscles are elevated and retracted.

CLOSURE:

The temporal fascia is joined at the midline along the sagittal crest. Since the incisions curve laterally to follow the frontal crests, the temporal fascia is sutured to the loose fascia lying between the frontal crests. The frontalis, interscutularis, and occipitalis muscles are closed on the midline.

PLATE 2. APPROACH TO THE DORSOLATERAL SURFACE OF THE SKULL

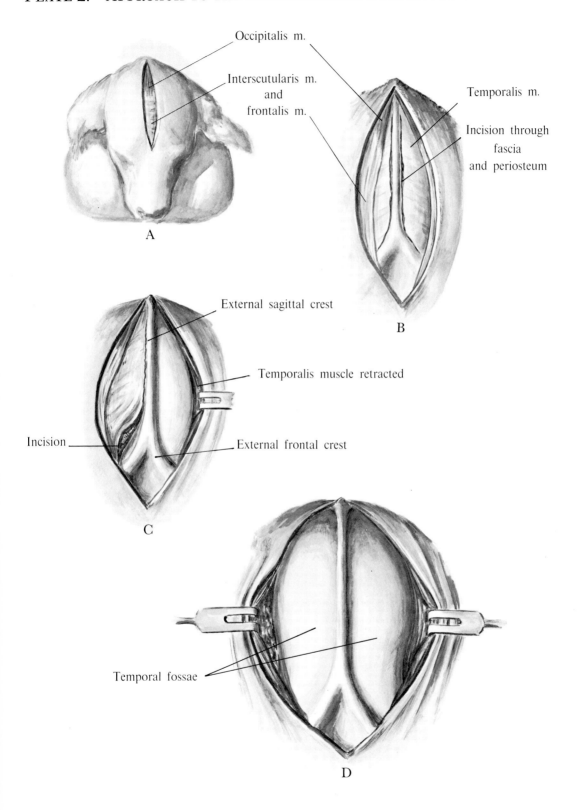

Occipitalis m.

Interscutularis m.
and
frontalis m.

Temporalis m.

Incision through
fascia
and periosteum

A

B

External sagittal crest

Temporalis muscle retracted

Incision

External frontal crest

C

Temporal fossae

D

APPROACH TO THE CAUDAL SURFACE OF THE SKULL

INDICATIONS:

1. Open reduction of fractures of the occipital bone.

2. Exposure of the caudal portion of the cerebellum and the cranial portion of the brain stem.

DESCRIPTION OF PROCEDURE:

A. The midline portion of the skin incision extends caudally from the external occipital protuberance about one third the length of the neck. The transverse incision follows the nuchal line of the occiput and ends just short of the base of the ears.

The subcutaneous fascia is incised in the same lines as the skin and is undermined with the skin to allow lateral retraction of each skin flap. The platysma muscle will be incised and retracted with subcutaneous fascia.

B. The first muscle seen upon retraction of the skin is the superficial cervicoauricularis. Originating on the exposed area of the cervical midline and passing cranially toward the ears, this muscle resembles a chevron with the point situated caudally. The muscle is incised on the midline and each muscle belly allowed to retract cranially. The temporal muscles, the external occipital protuberance, and the dorsal cervical muscles inserting on the occiput can now be visualized.

C. The dorsal muscle mass is transected close to the insertion on the nuchal line of the occiput. The use of electrocautery for this cutting is very helpful in minimizing hemorrhage. Enough tissue is left on the occiput to allow re-suturing of the muscles.

CLOSURE:

The cervical muscles are attached to the occiput by using mattress sutures which engage the fibrous muscle insertions remaining on the bone. The external sheath of the temporal muscles may also be utilized to securely anchor these sutures.

COMMENTS:

The caudal brain stem and cranial spinal cord may be exposed by elevating the muscles from the atlas and performing a dorsal laminectomy on this vertebra.

Page 16

PLATE 3. APPROACH TO THE CAUDAL SURFACE OF THE SKULL

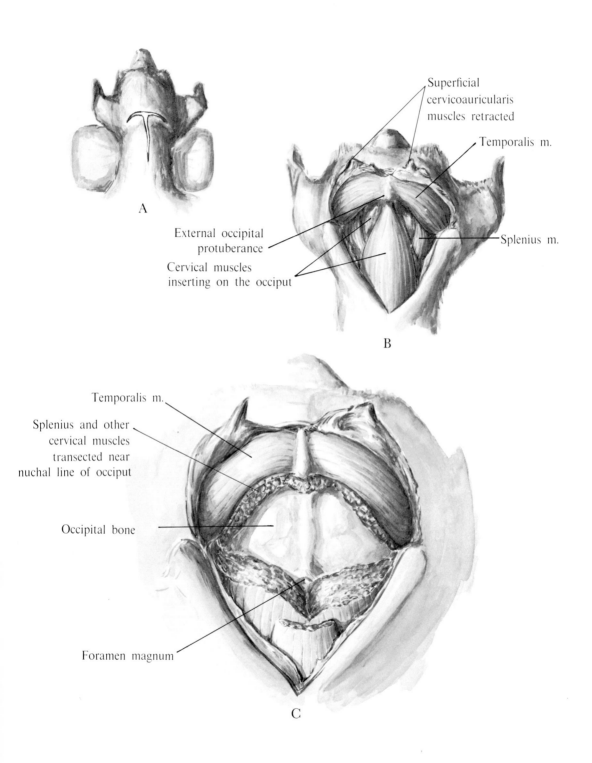

A

Superficial
cervicoauricularis
muscles retracted

Temporalis m.

External occipital
protuberance

Cervical muscles
inserting on the occiput

Splenius m.

B

Temporalis m.

Splenius and other
cervical muscles
transected near
nuchal line of occiput

Occipital bone

Foramen magnum

C

III | THE VERTEBRAL COLUMN

APPROACH TO THE CERVICAL VERTEBRAE AND INTER-VERTEBRAL DISCS THROUGH A VENTRAL INCISION

INDICATION:

Fenestration and curettage of intervertebral discs.

DESCRIPTION OF PROCEDURE:

A. The animal, with tracheal catheter in place, is secured in the supine position. A sandbag is placed under the neck to cause definite extension of the cervical vertebral column. The skin incision extends from the manubrium to the larynx.

B. The incision is deepened by midline separation of the paired bellies of the sternomastoideus and underlying sternohyoideus muscles.

Lateral retraction of these muscles exposes the trachea, esophagus, deep cervical fascia, and the carotid sheath.

C. Left lateral retraction of the trachea and esophagus allows blunt dissection through the deep cervical fascia to the longus colli muscle, which covers the ventral surfaces of the cervical vertebrae. The midline ventral processes of the vertebrae can be palpated through this muscle.

PLATE 4. APPROACH TO THE CERVICAL VERTEBRAE AND INTERVERTEBRAL DISCS THROUGH A VENTRAL INCISION

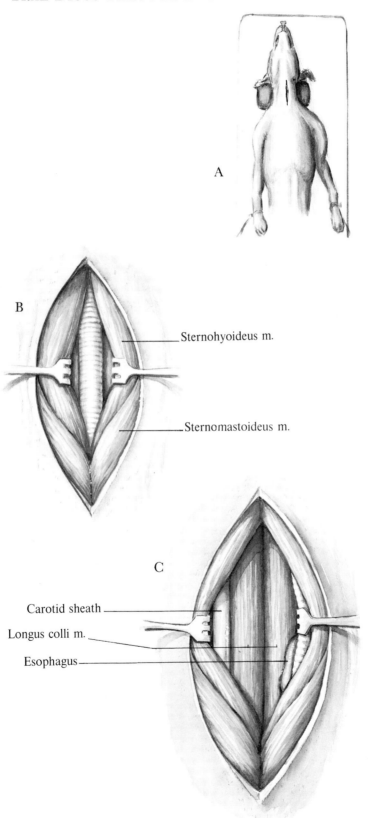

A

B — Sternohyoideus m.

Sternomastoideus m.

C

Carotid sheath

Longus colli m.

Esophagus

D. Longitudinal separation of longus colli muscle fibers overlying each ventral process exposes the aponeurosis of the muscle on the process. By working caudally from the eminence of the process, the tendon is gently scraped from the bone until the ventral longitudinal ligament is exposed. The exact location of the intervertebral space is identified by exploration with a 22-gauge needle, which is walked off the process caudally until it penetrates the ventral longitudinal ligament and the annulus fibrosus of the disc.

E. Fenestration is accomplished by a stab incision through the ventral longitudinal ligament and the annulus fibrosus. This opening into the disc may have to be enlarged for disc curettage.

CLOSURE:

The deep fascia is not sutured. The sternohyoideus and mastoideus muscles are closed along the midline, and the subcutaneous fascia is likewise united.

COMMENTS:

Care must be used in the retraction of tissues to avoid damage to the carotid sheath, the esophagus and trachea, and the right recurrent laryngeal nerve, which lies on the dorsolateral aspect of the trachea. The location of a specific intervertebral space is determined by first identifying the caudal borders of the wings of the atlas by palpation. The ventral midline process which lies on a line directly between the wings is the process of the atlas (C 1). Other processes can then be numbered by counting caudally from C 1.

PLATE 5. APPROACH TO THE CERVICAL VERTEBRAE AND INTER-VERTEBRAL DISCS THROUGH A VENTRAL INCISION—*Continued*

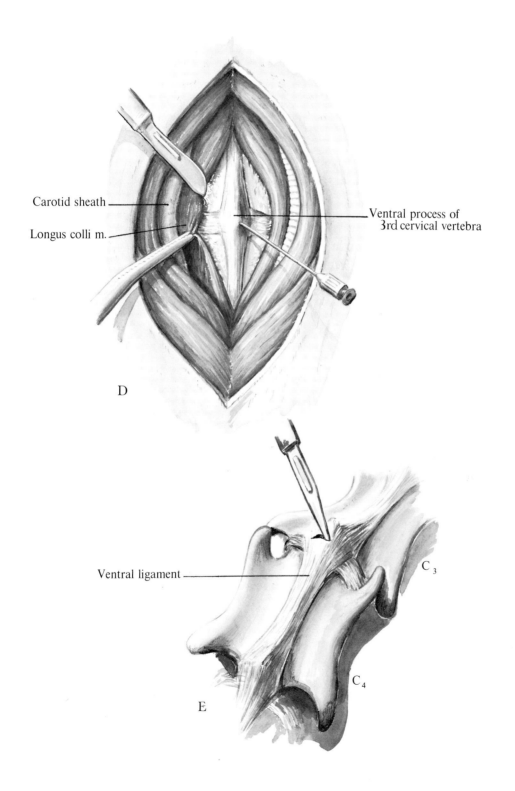

Carotid sheath

Longus colli m.

Ventral process of 3rd cervical vertebra

D

Ventral ligament

C₃

C₄

E

APPROACH TO THE CERVICAL VERTEBRAE THROUGH A DORSAL INCISION

INDICATIONS:

   1. Open reduction of fractures and luxations of the vertebrae.
   2. Dorsal laminectomy.

DESCRIPTION OF PROCEDURE:

A. The animal is positioned in sternal recumbency with a sandbag placed under the neck to elevate it and to cause flexion of the cervical spine. A tracheal catheter is imperative to maintain a patent airway in this position.

The midline skin incision extends from the external occipital protuberance to the first thoracic vertebra.

B. As the subcutaneous fascia is incised and the skin margins retracted, the almost transparent fibrous aponeurosis of the platysma muscle comes into view.

An incision is now made through the median fibrous raphe. This incision is deepened until the nuchal ligament is exposed.

C. The dorsolateral cervical muscles separated by this incision are retracted laterally to expose the nuchal ligament. The spinous processes can now be palpated under the ligament.

An incision is made in the rectus capitis, spinalis et semispinalis cervicis, and multifidus muscles along one side of the nuchal ligament. The incision is deepened along the lateral side of the spinous processes to the vertebral arch.

D. Elevation and retraction of the muscles from the vertebrae is done first on the side that was incised. This is best accomplished with a periosteal elevator or with the blunt end of the scalpel handle. The insertion of the nuchal ligament is now elevated from the spinous process of the axis and the entire ligament is retracted with the muscles on the side opposite the incision. The ligament thus remains firmly attached to the muscles of one side.

Lateral elevation of the muscles from the vertebral arch should be kept to a minimum since rather large branches of the vertebral artery course through the muscles near each articular process. Elevation of muscles beyond the articular processes will result in excessive hemorrhage.

CLOSURE:

The nuchal ligament is secured to the axis by two sutures of 26 gauge monofilament stainless wire. These wires are passed through holes drilled transversely through the spinous process of the axis.

The external fascia of the deep muscles can now be sutured to the nuchal ligament. The median fibrous raphe is closed next, followed by the subcutaneous fascia.

PLATE 6. APPROACH TO THE CERVICAL VERTEBRAE THROUGH A DORSAL INCISION

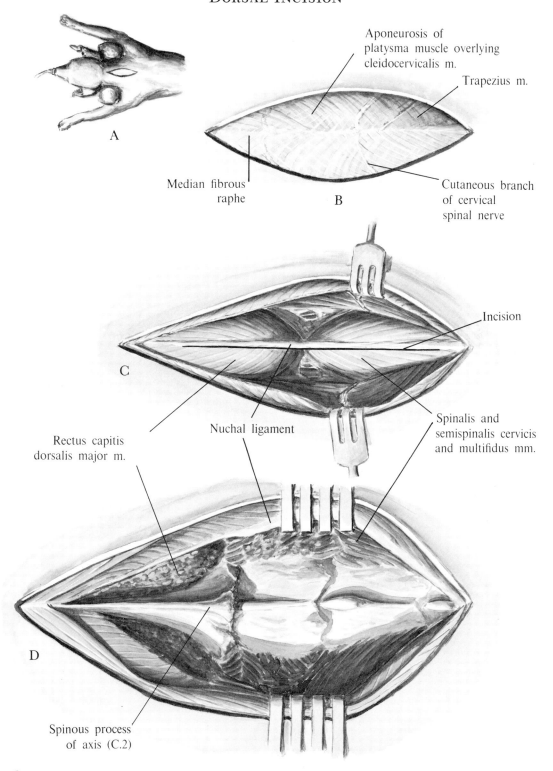

A

Aponeurosis of
platysma muscle overlying
cleidocervicalis m.

Trapezius m.

Median fibrous
raphe

B

Cutaneous branch
of cervical
spinal nerve

Incision

C

Rectus capitis
dorsalis major m.

Nuchal ligament

Spinalis and
semispinalis cervicis
and multifidus mm.

D

Spinous process
of axis (C.2)

COMMENTS:

If the spinous process of the axis has been removed in the course of laminectomy, the nuchal ligament is secured to the rectus capitis muscle by mattress sutures that bite deeply into this muscle.

APPROACH TO THE THORACOLUMBAR VERTEBRAE AND INTERVERTEBRAL DISCS THROUGH A DORSAL INCISION

INDICATIONS:

1. Open reduction of fractures and luxations of the vertebrae.
2. Dorsal laminectomy and hemilaminectomy.
3. Fenestration and curettage of intervertebral discs T 9–10 through L 6–7.

EXPLANATORY NOTE:

The exposure for hemilaminectomy and for fenestration and curettage is usually unilateral. The procedure is as described below in paragraphs A through C. The incision in the supraspinous ligament (illustration C) is made only on the side to be exposed, and the muscles are then elevated on that side.

DESCRIPTION OF PROCEDURE:

A. The length of the dorsal midline incision is determined by the number of vertebrae that are to be exposed. In order to obtain sufficient muscle retraction it is necessary to extend the incision the length of two vertebrae cranial and caudal to the vertebra in question. The incision shown here centers on L 1 and extends from T 12 to L 3.

B. Subcutaneous fat and fascia are incised until the dense lumbodorsal fascia is reached. The fat is undermined to free it from the fascia and to allow its retraction with the skin.

C. The supraspinous ligament is incised around the tip of each spinous process and between each process. The incision is continued down to the vertebral arch between each process to complete the midline muscle separation.

D. The multifidus lumborum muscle is bluntly elevated from the spinous processes and vertebral arches laterally to the mammillary processes. This is sufficient exposure for a dorsal laminectomy that is to be limited to the width of the vertebral arch between the articular processes.

E. For an extensive dorsal laminectomy ("deroofing" of the vertebral arch) and for fenestration and curettage, muscular elevation must be continued laterally and ventrally to the level of the transverse processes and the ribs.

The muscular aponeurosis on each mammillary and accessory process must be incised to free it from the process. A small arterial bleeder will be encountered and severed at each process.

An attempt is made to leave intact the dorsal branches of the spinal nerves that emerge from the intervertebral foramina immediately ventral to each accessory process.

CLOSURE:

The lumbodorsal fascia is sutured over the tips of the spinous processes. The subcutaneous fat and fascia are closed with a second layer of sutures.

PLATE 7. APPROACH TO THE THORACOLUMBAR VERTEBRAE AND INTERVERTEBRAL DISCS THROUGH A DORSAL INCISION

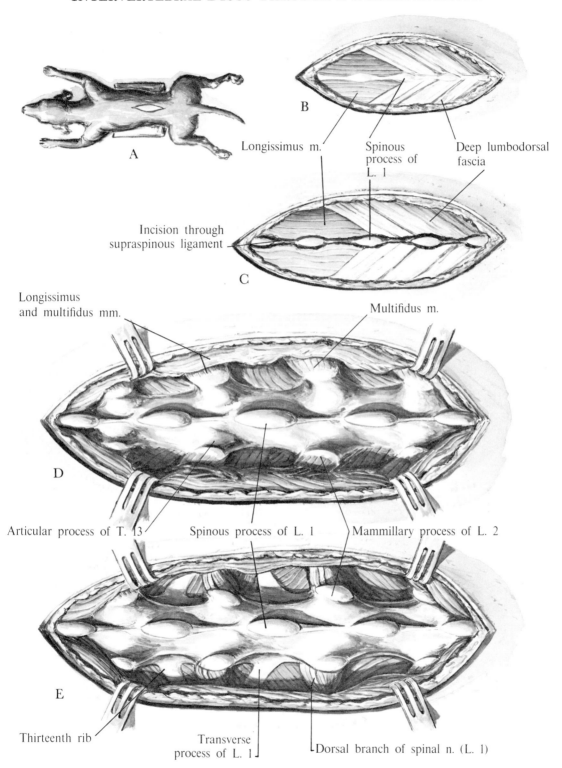

A

B

Longissimus m.

Spinous process of L. 1

Deep lumbodorsal fascia

Incision through supraspinous ligament

C

Longissimus and multifidus mm.

Multifidus m.

D

Articular process of T. 13

Spinous process of L. 1

Mammillary process of L. 2

E

Thirteenth rib

Transverse process of L. 1

Dorsal branch of spinal n. (L. 1)

COMMENTS:

A moderately tight elastic bandage is applied around the trunk for 72 hours to prevent subcutaneous serum accumulation.

APPROACH TO THE THORACOLUMBAR INTERVERTEBRAL DISCS THROUGH AN INTERCOSTAL INCISION

INDICATION:

Fenestration and curettage of intervertebral discs T 10–11 through L 1–2.

DESCRIPTION OF PROCEDURE:

A. The skin incision is made in the intercostal space immediately cranial to the disc to be exposed, for example, for the disc at T 11–12, the incision is made at intercostal space T 10–11. The two lumbar discs may be reached by an incision at space T 12–13. The incision extends from the level of the lateral border of the iliocostalis lumborum muscle to the costochondral junction.

B. Subcutaneous fat and fascia, intercostal muscles, and parietal pleura are all incised midway between the adjacent ribs. The serratus dorsalis muscle will also be encountered in all spaces except T 10–11. The ribs are firmly retracted to provide access to the thoracic cavity. The diaphragmatic lobe of the lung is packed off to allow more working room.

C. The sympathetic nerve trunk lying dorsolateral to the aorta is mobilized sufficiently to allow retraction ventrally. The quadratus lumborum muscle will be found originating from the bodies of the last three thoracic vertebrae.

D. The quadratus muscle is elevated slightly to allow lateral retraction. The aorta may be gently retracted ventrally, but this is seldom required since the aorta stays toward the lower side owing to its own weight. An incision is made through the ventral longitudinal ligament and the annulus fibrosus after locating the disc by probing with a needle 3 to 4 mm. cranial to the rib. The disc is now ready for curettage.

CLOSURE:

Adjacent ribs are encircled by three or four sutures of size 1 extra chromic catgut. The sutures are placed but not tied until the ribs are squeezed together sufficiently to appose the incised intercostal muscles. The rest of the tissues are closed in layers.

COMMENTS:

The aorta is best protected with the tip of a finger during curettage. Lumbar discs L 1–2 and L 2–3 are exposed by a skin incision at intercostal space T 12–13 and an incision of the crus of the diaphragm.

Page 28

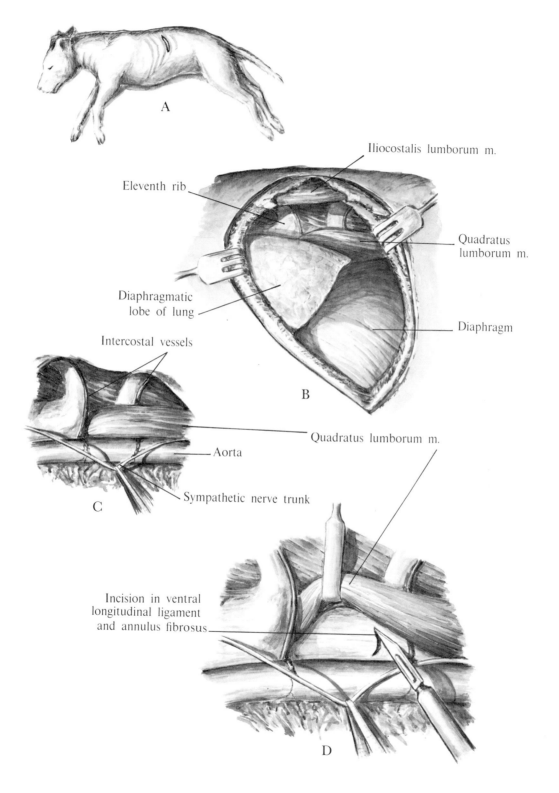

A

Iliocostalis lumborum m.

Eleventh rib

Quadratus
lumborum m.

Diaphragmatic
lobe of lung

Diaphragm

Intercostal vessels

B

Quadratus lumborum m.

Aorta

Sympathetic nerve trunk

C

Incision in ventral
longitudinal ligament
and annulus fibrosus

D

Page 29

APPROACH TO THE SACROCOCCYGEAL VERTEBRAE

INDICATION:

Open reduction of fractures and luxations of the sacrum and cranial coccygeal vertebrae.

DESCRIPTION OF PROCEDURE:

A. The dorsal process of the seventh lumbar vertebra marks the cranial end of the skin incision, which then extends caudally to a point between the tubera ischii.

The subcutaneous fat is often quite thick in this area. It is incised on the midline and undermined to allow its retraction with the skin.

B. The deep fascia is incised on the midline between the paired bellies of the medial sacrococcygeal muscles. The incision is deepened through the intermuscular septum until the median sacral crest is reached.

C. The medial sacrococcygeal muscles are elevated (by sharp and blunt dissection) from the dorsal surface of the sacrum and coccygeal vertebrae and are retracted laterally.

The lateral limits of muscular elevation are marked by the mammilloarticular processes of the sacrum. Just lateral to these processes are the dorsal sacral foramina, through which pass the dorsal divisions of the sacral nerves and vessels.

CLOSURE:

A row of sutures is placed in the deep fascia and a second row in the subcutaneous fat and fascia.

PLATE 9. APPROACH TO THE SACROCOCCYGEAL VERTEBRAE

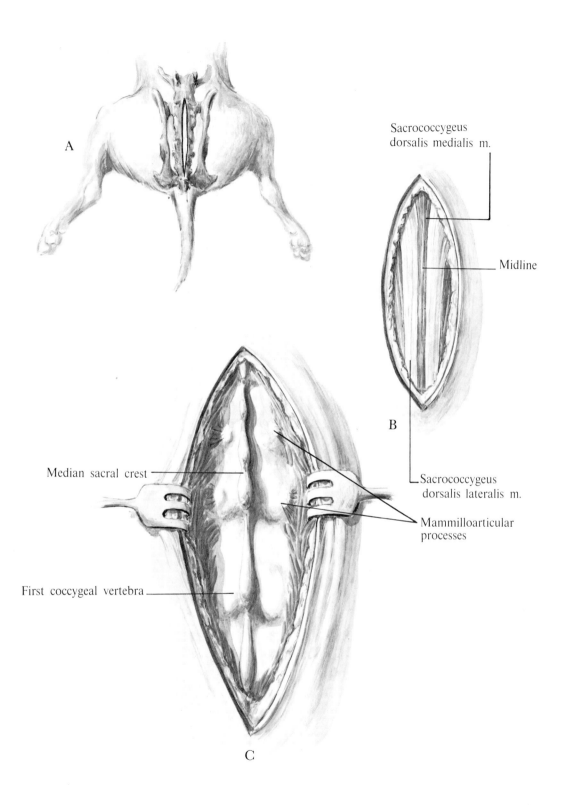

A

Sacrococcygeus
dorsalis medialis m.

Midline

B

Sacrococcygeus
dorsalis lateralis m.

Median sacral crest

Mammilloarticular
processes

First coccygeal vertebra

C

APPROACH TO THE COCCYGEAL VERTEBRAE

INDICATIONS:

1. Open reduction of fractures and luxations of the vertebrae.
2. Treatment of malunion of fractures or congenital malformation of the vertebrae by osteotomy.

DESCRIPTION OF PROCEDURE:

A. The skin and subcutaneous fascial incision is made along the dorsal midline of the tail and extends the length of one vertebra proximal and distal to the vertebra to be exposed.

B. Undermining and retraction of the skin margins reveals the sacrococcygeal muscles under a layer of deep fascia. This fascia is incised on the midline between the paired medial sacrococcygeal muscles. The incision is continued into the intermuscular septum until the dorsal surface of the vertebrae is reached.

C. A combination of sharp and blunt dissection is used to elevate the muscles from the vertebrae.

CLOSURE:

Deep and subcutaneous fascia are closed in one layer of sutures.

COMMENTS:

Only by working close to the bone during the muscular elevation can the dorsal lateral coccygeal artery and dorsal coccygeal nerve trunk be avoided.

The tail should be bandaged to minimize movement as much as possible for four to five days postoperatively.

PLATE 10. APPROACH TO THE COCCYGEAL VERTEBRAE

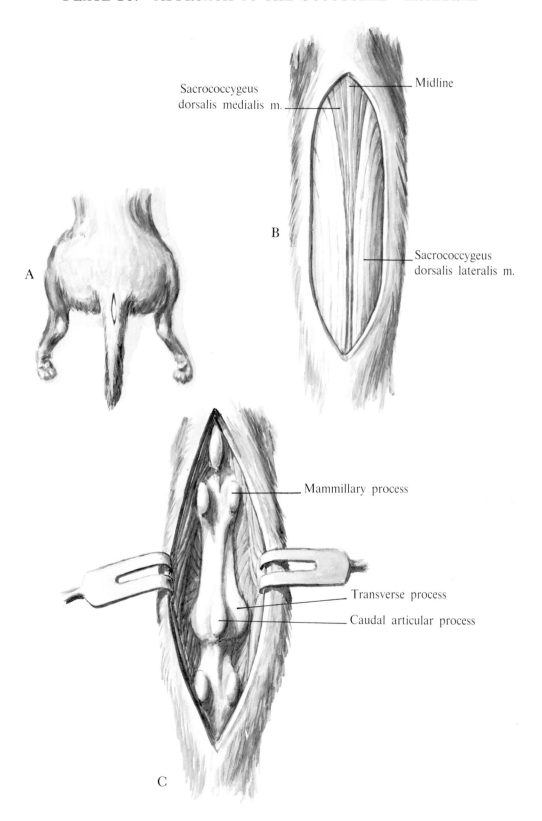

Sacrococcygeus dorsalis medialis m.

Midline

B

Sacrococcygeus dorsalis lateralis m.

A

Mammillary process

Transverse process

Caudal articular process

C

IV | THE FORELIMB

APPROACH TO THE BODY OF THE SCAPULA

INDICATION:

Open reduction of fractures of the body that extend into the glenoid cavity.

DESCRIPTION OF PROCEDURE:

A. The skin and subcutaneous fascial incision is made directly on the spine of the scapula. The skin and fascia are retracted following the undermining of the edges of the incision.

B. An incision is now made in the deep fascia along the spine of the scapula and is deepened to free the origins of the deltoid and omotransversarius muscles and the insertion of the trapezius muscle. These muscles are undermined and allowed to retract sufficiently to expose the spine and the deep spinatus muscles.

C. The spinatus muscles are elevated subperiosteally from their attachments on the spine of the scapula. The bellies of the muscles can then be bluntly undermined and retracted from the body of the scapula.

CLOSURE:

A single row of sutures will suffice to close all the incised structures. The suture line runs directly along the spine and includes the deep fascia and the external sheath of the spinatus muscles.

COMMENTS:

Elevation of the infraspinatus muscle from the scapular spine is complicated by the presence of the metacromion in the *cat*. This protuberance, located on the spine 1 to 2 cm. proximal to the acromion, overhangs the infraspinatus slightly, but it does not actually alter the procedure.

PLATE 11. APPROACH TO THE BODY OF THE SCAPULA

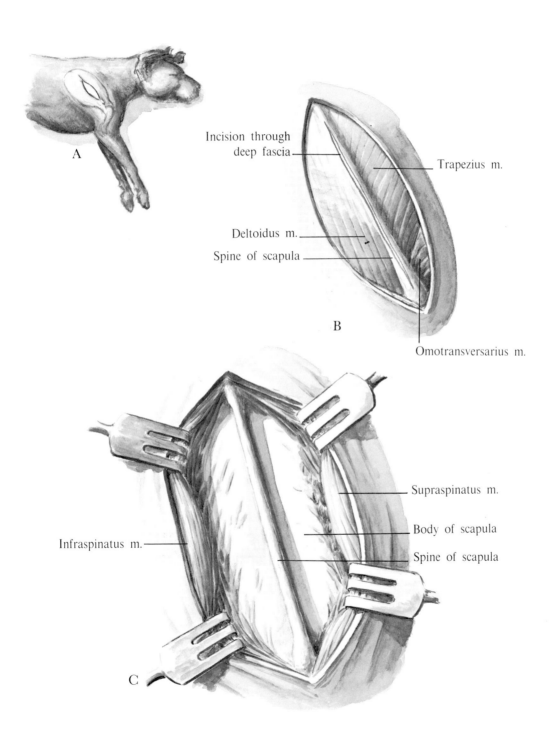

A

Incision through deep fascia

Trapezius m.

Deltoidus m.

Spine of scapula

B

Omotransversarius m.

Supraspinatus m.

Body of scapula

Spine of scapula

Infraspinatus m.

C

Page 37

APPROACH TO THE SHOULDER JOINT AND DISTAL END OF THE SCAPULA

INDICATIONS:

1. Open reduction of fractures of the articular angle of the scapula.
2. Open reduction of chronic luxations of the shoulder joint.
3. Removal of loose bodies in the joint.

DESCRIPTION OF PROCEDURE:

A. The curved incision begins at the middle of the scapula and follows the spine distally, crossing the joint and continuing over the lateral surface of the humerus to the midpoint of the shaft.

B. The skin margins are undermined and retracted after the subcutaneous fascia and fat are incised in the same line as the skin incision.

An incision is made in the deep fascia directly over the spine of the scapula and is deepened to free the origin of the spinous part of the deltoid and the omotransversarius muscles and the insertion of the trapezius muscle on the spine. The incision is continued distally through the deep fascia directly over the acromial part of the deltoid and is halted before it reaches the cephalic vein. The incised fascia is undermined and retracted from the acromial part of the deltoid.

C. The omotransversarius and trapezius are undermined and allowed to retract cranially. The division between the two parts of the deltoid muscle is developed by blunt dissection to allow freeing of the spinous part of the muscle and its caudal retraction with the deep fascia. The acromion is osteotomized to include all of the origin of the acromial part of the deltoid. A 6 mm. osteotome is used for this division.

PLATE 12. APPROACH TO THE SHOULDER JOINT AND DISTAL END
OF THE SCAPULA

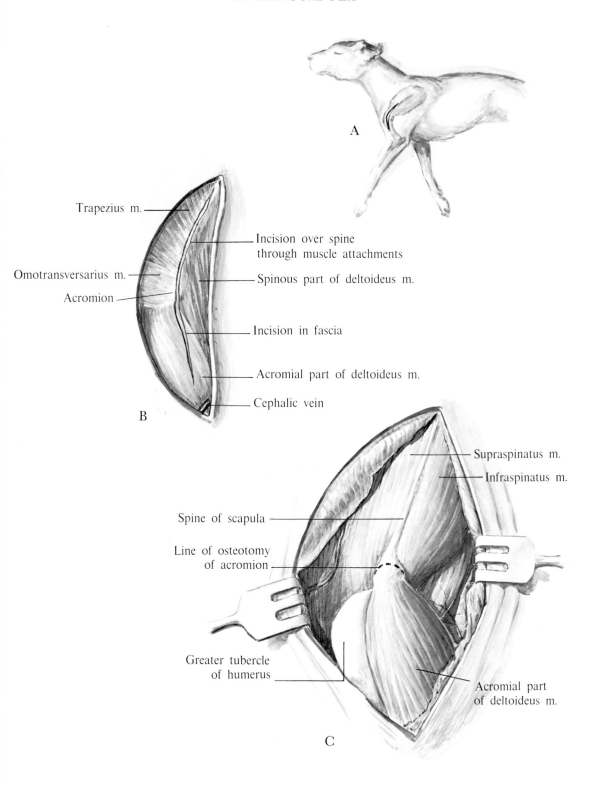

A

Trapezius m.

Incision over spine
through muscle attachments

Spinous part of deltoideus m.

Omotransversarius m.

Acromion

Incision in fascia

Acromial part of deltoideus m.

Cephalic vein

B

Supraspinatus m.

Infraspinatus m.

Spine of scapula

Line of osteotomy
of acromion

Greater tubercle
of humerus

Acromial part
of deltoideus m.

C

Page 39

D. It is now possible to free the acromial part of the deltoid from the shaft of the humerus and to reflect it distally, while its insertion is left on the deltoid tuberosity undisturbed.

The supraspinatus and infraspinatus muscles are bluntly elevated from the spine and body of the scapula sufficiently to allow their retraction as shown. Note the position of the suprascapular nerve in illustration E and avoid this structure during the elevation and retraction of the infraspinatus.

E. Exposure of the joint requires tenotomy of the infraspinatus muscle. This cut is made near the muscle's insertion on the humerus, with enough stump being left to receive one or two sutures. In some cases it may be necessary to treat the teres minor muscle in a like manner, thus allowing greater exposure of the ventrolateral aspect of the joint capsule.

CLOSURE:

Mattress sutures are used to join the severed infraspinatus. The acromion is attached to the spine by two 26 gauge monofilament stainless steel sutures placed through holes drilled in the bones. A single tier of sutures may be used to close the remaining muscles and deep fascia. Starting at the proximal end of the incision the stitch engages the deep fascia, the trapezius, the external sheath of both spinatus muscles, the spinous part of the deltoid, and the deep fascia. This pattern is continued distally, with the omotransversarius replacing the trapezius as the acromion is approached. Distal to the acromion the deep fascia alone is closed.

COMMENTS

Elevation of the infraspinatus muscle from the scapular spine is complicated by the presence of the metacromion in the *cat*. This protuberance, located 1 to 2 cm. proximal to the acromion, overhangs the infraspinatus slightly, but it does not actually alter the procedure.

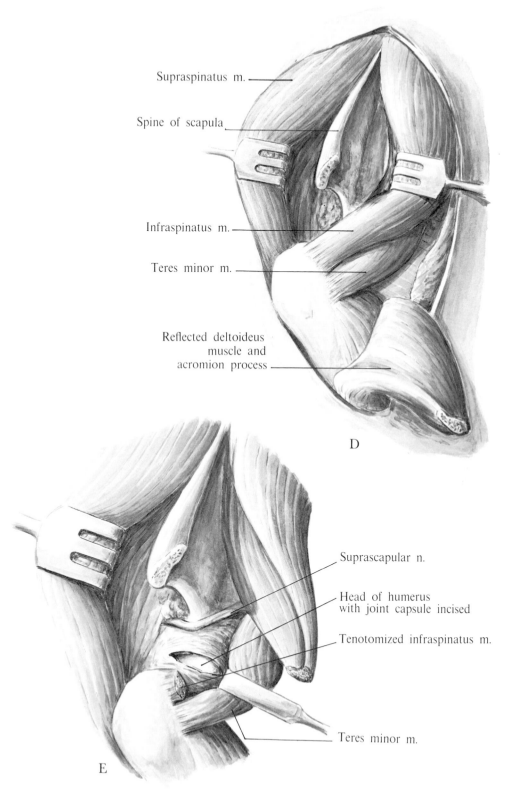

Supraspinatus m.

Spine of scapula

Infraspinatus m.

Teres minor m.

Reflected deltoideus
muscle and
acromion process

D

Suprascapular n.

Head of humerus
with joint capsule incised

Tenotomized infraspinatus m.

Teres minor m.

E

Page 41

APPROACH TO THE PROXIMAL SHAFT OF THE HUMERUS

INDICATIONS:

1. Open reduction of fractures of the proximal half of the shaft of the humerus.
2. Open reduction of epiphyseal fractures of the head of the humerus.

DESCRIPTION OF PROCEDURE:

A. The skin incision is made slightly lateral to the cranial midline of the bone and extends from the greater tubercle of the humerus proximally to a point near the midshaft of the bone.

B. Following the undermining and retraction of the skin, an incision is made through the deep fascia along the caudal border of the brachiocephalicus muscle.

C. The brachiocephalicus can be retracted cranially following blunt dissection between the muscle and the bone. An incision is made through the periosteum between the cranial border of the deltoideus muscle and the deep pectoral muscle. Several branches of the distal communicating vein will be severed by this incision and must be ligated.

D. Exposure of the shaft is accomplished by the subperiosteal elevation of the deep pectoral and deltoideus muscles. This elevation will usually also include a portion of the origin of the lateral head of the triceps, which lies under the deltoideus.

CLOSURE:

The periosteal and deep fascial incision may be closed in one layer.

PLATE 14. APPROACH TO THE PROXIMAL SHAFT OF THE HUMERUS

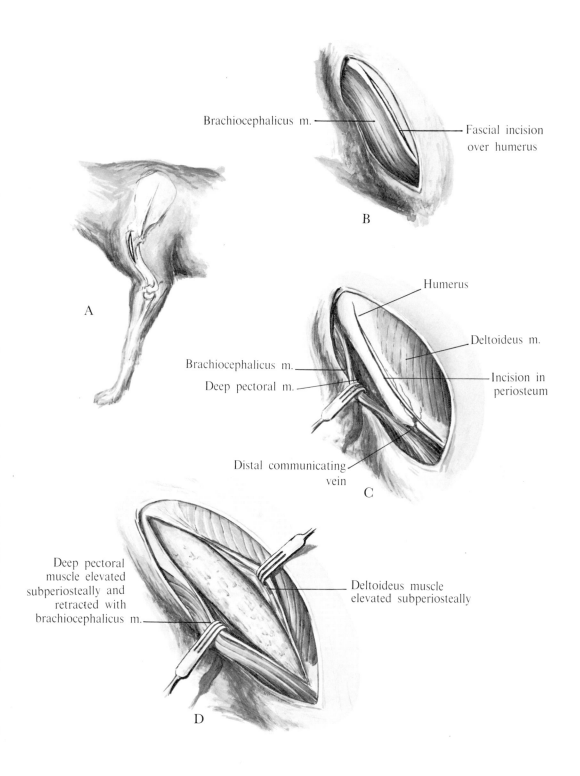

Brachiocephalicus m.

Fascial incision
over humerus

B

A

Humerus

Deltoideus m.

Brachiocephalicus m.

Deep pectoral m.

Incision in
periosteum

Distal communicating
vein

C

Deep pectoral
muscle elevated
subperiosteally and
retracted with
brachiocephalicus m.

Deltoideus muscle
elevated subperiosteally

D

Page 43

APPROACH TO THE DISTAL SHAFT OF THE HUMERUS THROUGH A LATERAL INCISION

INDICATION:

Open reduction of fractures between the midshaft and the supracondylar area of the humerus.

DESCRIPTION OF PROCEDURE:

A. The craniolateral border of the humerus is the guide for this incision, which commences at the midshaft and ends at the lateral epicondyle.

B. The skin margins are mobilized and retracted. Subcutaneous fascia and fat are incised in the same line as the skin, with the cephalic vein, which will cross the proximal end of the incision, being avoided. The deep fascia of the brachium is incised along the cranial border of the triceps. The incision curves caudally, parallel to the cephalic vein, to allow mobilization of the vein. The radial nerve must be protected when the distal end of this incision is opened.

C. The deep fascia is undermined to allow cranial retraction of the cephalic vein and exposure of the radial nerve. An incision is made in the intermuscular septum between the brachialis and the brachiocephalicus muscles.

D. The brachiocephalicus and the distal portions of the superficial pectoral muscle are elevated at their insertions on the humerus as necessary to allow cranial retraction. The brachialis is freed from the bone by blunt dissection and is retracted caudally with the triceps and the radial nerve. To obtain better exposure of the distal portion of the bone, the lateral head of the triceps muscle can be retracted caudally and the brachialis muscle and radial nerve retracted cranially.

CLOSURE:

The deep fascia is closed in one layer.

COMMENTS:

Great care must be taken at all times to protect the radial nerve. The medial approach (Plate 16) is preferred for supracondylar fractures, since the exposure is much better.

PLATE 15. APPROACH TO THE DISTAL SHAFT OF THE HUMERUS THROUGH A LATERAL INCISION

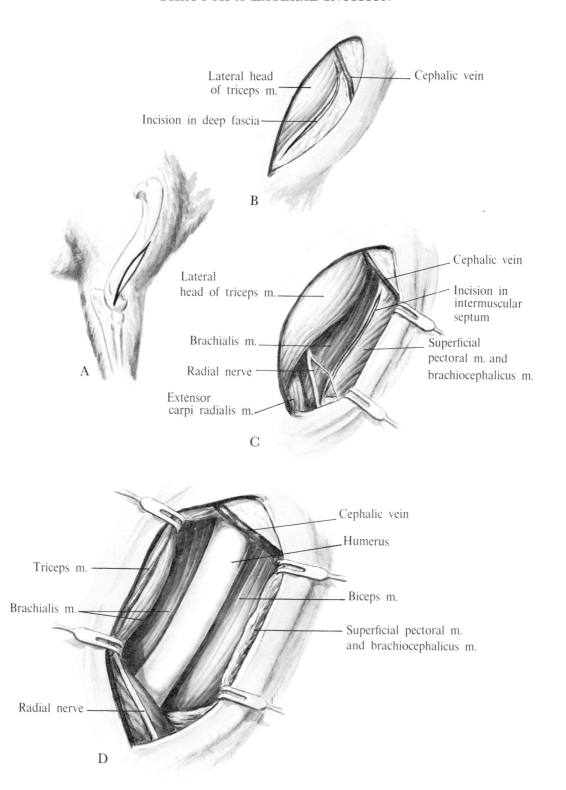

Lateral head of triceps m.

Cephalic vein

Incision in deep fascia

B

Lateral head of triceps m.

Cephalic vein

Incision in intermuscular septum

Brachialis m.

Radial nerve

Extensor carpi radialis m.

Superficial pectoral m. and brachiocephalicus m.

A

C

Cephalic vein

Humerus

Triceps m.

Brachialis m.

Biceps m.

Superficial pectoral m. and brachiocephalicus m.

Radial nerve

D

Page 45

APPROACH TO THE DISTAL SHAFT OF THE HUMERUS
THROUGH A MEDIAL INCISION

INDICATION:

Open reduction of fractures on the supracondylar portion of the humerus.

DESCRIPTION OF PROCEDURE:

A. The skin incision extends from the medial epicondyle proximally along the cranial border of the humerus to the midshaft of the bone.

B. The skin is undermined and the subcutaneous fat is elevated sufficiently to allow visualization of the brachial and collateral ulnar vessels. The ulnar and median nerves which accompany these vessels are not yet visible; they lie slightly deeper. An incision is made in the deep fascia directly over the distal shaft of the humerus and between the blood vessels. It may be necessary to continue the incision proximally over the vessels.

C. Blunt dissection of the subfascial fat will expose the underlying structures. The manner in which the brachial vessels and the median nerve are mobilized depends on the area of the bone that is to be exposed. The method illustrated here is used when the extreme distal portion of the bone is involved. If the proximal portion of the exposed area is of more interest, these vessels and nerves may be freed and retracted caudally with the triceps and the collateral ulnar vessels.

D. The biceps and triceps muscles are elevated from the shaft of the bone. The periosteal branches of blood vessels are ligated as required. Subperiosteal elevation of a portion of the insertion of the superficial pectoral and brachiocephalicus muscles is necessary to fully expose the cranial surface of the bone.

E. The *cat* shows a marked difference from the dog in this area. Note the supracondylar foramen in the bone through which the median nerve passes. Note also the short head of the medial triceps running caudal to the medial condyle and inserting on the medial side of the olecranon. The ulnar nerve passes under this muscle.

CLOSURE:

The deep fascia is closed to hold the muscles in place.

COMMENTS:

This approach is preferred over the lateral approach (Plate 15) for exposure of the supracondylar area. In the lateral approach this area of the humerus is obscured by the origins of the extensors of the antebrachium on the lateral epicondyle.

Page 46

PLATE 16. APPROACH TO THE DISTAL SHAFT OF THE HUMERUS THROUGH A MEDIAL INCISION

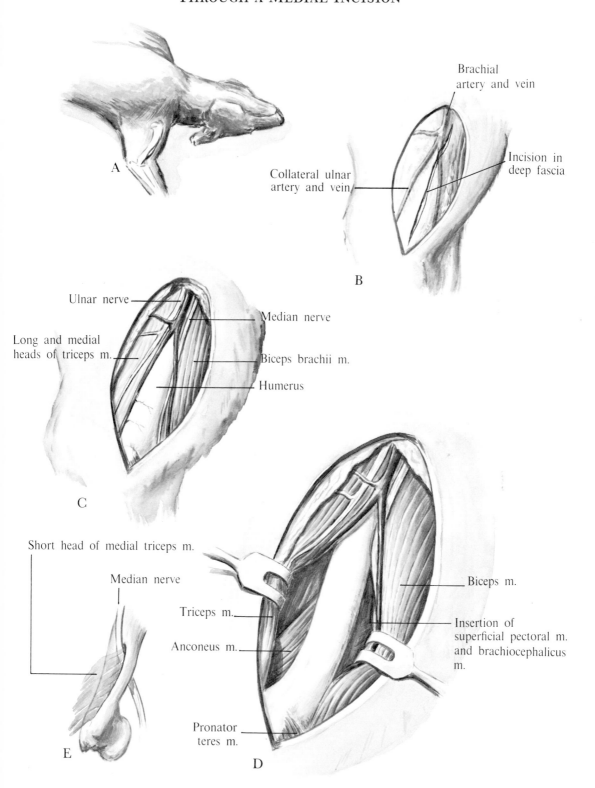

A

Brachial
artery and vein

Collateral ulnar
artery and vein

Incision in
deep fascia

B

Ulnar nerve

Median nerve

Long and medial
heads of triceps m.

Biceps brachii m.

Humerus

C

Short head of medial triceps m.

Median nerve

Biceps m.

Triceps m.

Anconeus m.

Insertion of
superficial pectoral m.
and brachiocephalicus
m.

Pronator
teres m.

E

D

APPROACH TO THE MEDIAL CONDYLE OF THE HUMERUS

INDICATION:

Open reduction of fractures of the condyle.

DESCRIPTION OF PROCEDURE:

A.   The incision covers the lower fourth of the humerus, running parallel to the shaft and slightly caudal to the medial epicondyle and ending distally just beyond the epicondyle. The subcutaneous fat and fascia are incised on the same line as the skin.

B.   The deep fascia is exposed following the undermining and retraction of the subcutaneous fascia and skin. The deep fascia is incised near the cranial border of the medial head of the triceps, with care being taken to avoid the underlying vessels and nerve.

C.   Elevation of the triceps reveals the ulnar nerve and the collateral ulnar vessels.

D.   The vessels and nerve are bluntly undermined and freed from the bone to allow their retraction with the triceps.

CLOSURE:

The deep and subcutaneous fascia can be closed in one suture tier.

PLATE 17. APPROACH TO THE MEDIAL CONDYLE OF THE HUMERUS

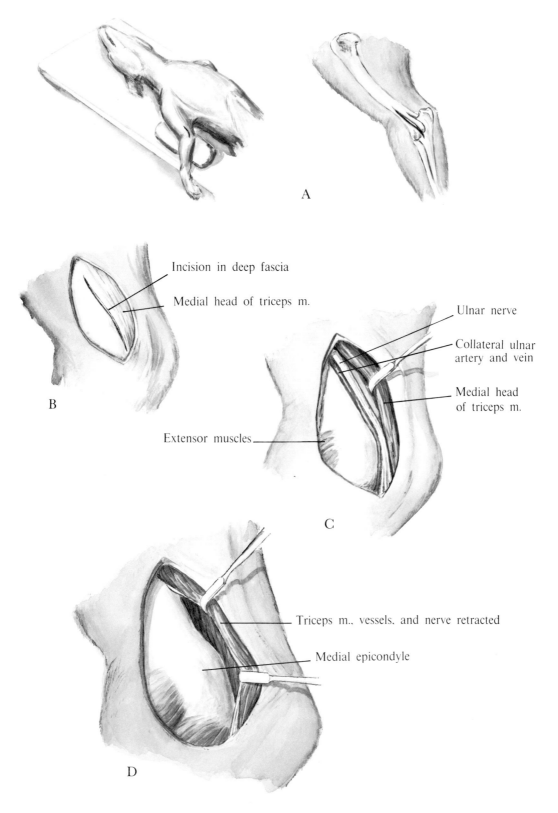

A

Incision in deep fascia

Medial head of triceps m.

B

Ulnar nerve

Collateral ulnar artery and vein

Medial head of triceps m.

Extensor muscles

C

Triceps m., vessels, and nerve retracted

Medial epicondyle

D

Page 49

APPROACH TO THE LATERAL CONDYLE
OF THE HUMERUS

INDICATION:

Open reduction of fractures of the condyle.

DESCRIPTION OF PROCEDURE:

A. The skin incision extends along the lower fourth of the humerus and crosses the joint to end distally on the ulna. The incision passes over or slightly caudal to the lateral epicondyle. The subcutaneous fascia is incised on the same line.

B. As the skin and subcutaneous fascia are retracted, the deep brachial fascia and the lateral head of the triceps muscle are exposed. An incision is made through the deep fascia near the cranial border of the triceps.

C. Bluntly undermining the triceps allows it to be retracted caudolaterally so that the condylar part of the humerus is exposed.

CLOSURE:

The deep and subcutaneous fascial incisions are closed separately.

COMMENTS:

The radial nerve passes between the brachialis muscle and the lateral head of the triceps just proximal to this incision. Some care should be exercised to avoid injury to this nerve when the deep fascial incision is made.

PLATE 18. APPROACH TO THE LATERAL CONDYLE OF THE HUMERUS

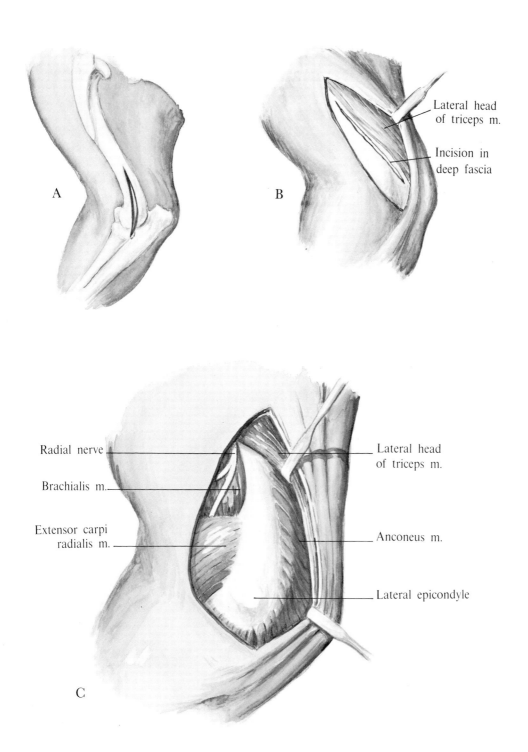

A

B

Lateral head
of triceps m.

Incision in
deep fascia

Radial nerve

Brachialis m.

Extensor carpi
radialis m.

Lateral head
of triceps m.

Anconeus m.

Lateral epicondyle

C

APPROACH TO THE ELBOW JOINT THROUGH A LATERAL INCISION

INDICATIONS

1. Open reduction of luxations of the elbow.
2. Removal of loose bodies from the caudal compartment of the joint.

EXPLANATORY NOTE:

This procedure is initiated as shown in illustrations A–C of Plate 18, Approach to the Lateral Condyle of the Humerus (p. 50).

DESCRIPTION OF PROCEDURE:

A.   With the lateral head of the triceps sufficiently undermined to allow its free caudal retraction, an incision is made through the anconeus muscle and the adherent joint capsule. The incision is made parallel to the humerus and midway between the humeral condyle and the olecranon.

B.   Reflection of the incised muscle exposes the joint space. Extreme flexion of the joint provides the best view of the interior of the joint.

CLOSURE:

Catgut sutures are placed in the anconeus muscle and joint capsule. The deep fascial incision is closed separately from that in the subcutaneous fascia.

COMMENTS:

This is the approach of choice for the removal of an ununited anconeal process.

PLATE 19. APPROACH TO THE ELBOW JOINT THROUGH A LATERAL INCISION

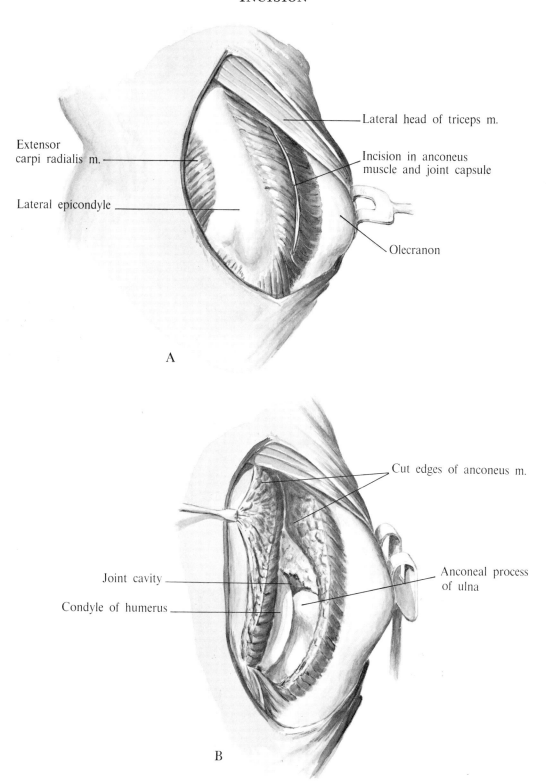

Lateral head of triceps m.

Extensor carpi radialis m.

Incision in anconeus muscle and joint capsule

Lateral epicondyle

Olecranon

A

Cut edges of anconeus m.

Joint cavity

Anconeal process of ulna

Condyle of humerus

B

Page 53

APPROACH TO THE ELBOW JOINT BY OSTEOTOMY
OF THE OLECRANON PROCESS

INDICATIONS:

1. Open reduction of comminuted fractures of the distal end of the humerus.
2. Open reduction of chronic luxations of the elbow joint.
3. Removal of loose bodies from the caudal compartment of the joint.

DESCRIPTION OF PROCEDURE:

A. A skin incision is made slightly lateral to the caudal midline of the leg. The incision extends from the distal third of the humerus to the proximal third of the ulna and crosses the elbow joint between the olecranon process and the lateral epicondyle.

B. Subcutaneous fat and deep fascia are incised to the muscle sheaths and then widely undermined to allow retraction of the cranial skin margin beyond the lateral epicondyle. The cranial border of the triceps is developed by blunt dissection and is undermined from the area of the lateral epicondyle to the olecranon.

C. The leg is elevated and the elbow flexed to allow dissection of the medial side of the joint.

D. The undermining of the deep fascia continues around the joint to the medial side until the caudal skin margin can be retracted beyond the medial epicondyle. The cranial border of the medial head of the triceps is undermined from the area of the medial condyle to the olecranon. The ulnar nerve and collateral ulnar vessels lie parallel to the cranial border of the medial head and deep to it, under the antebrachial fascia. The nerve and vessels should be identified and protected throughout the procedure by retracting them distally.

When operating on the *cat*, refer at this point to illustration E of Plate 16, Approach to the Distal Shaft of the Humerus Through a Medial Incision, (p. 47).

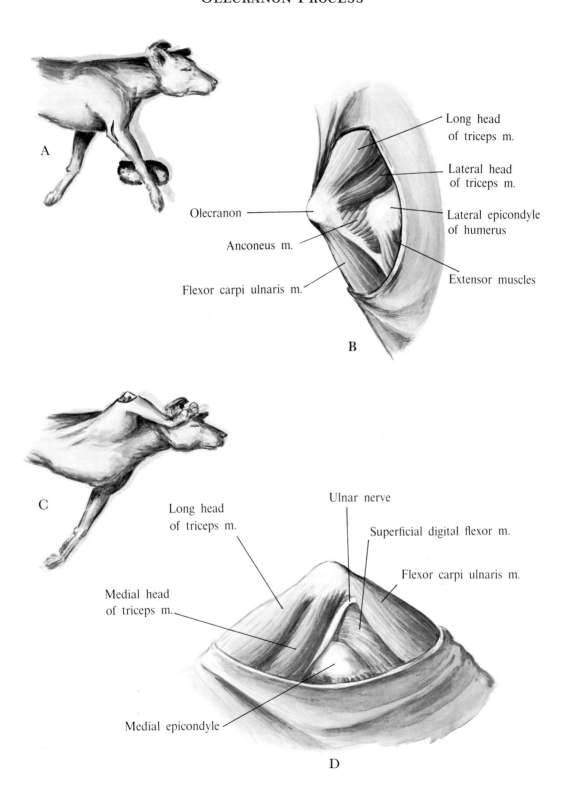

A

Long head
of triceps m.

Lateral head
of triceps m.

Olecranon

Lateral epicondyle
of humerus

Anconeus m.

Flexor carpi ulnaris m.

Extensor muscles

B

C

Ulnar nerve

Long head
of triceps m.

Superficial digital flexor m.

Flexor carpi ulnaris m.

Medial head
of triceps m.

Medial epicondyle

D

Page 55

APPROACH TO THE ELBOW JOINT BY OSTEOTOMY
OF THE OLECRANON PROCESS—*Continued*

E. The pilot hole for the bone screw used to reattach the olecranon process is best drilled before the osteotomy is done. In order to keep the drill in the medullary canal of the ulna, it is necessary to drill in a direction slightly lateral to the sagittal plane of the leg. Next a curved hemostat is used to pass the Gigli wire saw under the tendon of the triceps. The wire is positioned on the olecranon so as to include the entire insertion of the triceps tendon on the portion of bone to be cut free. The joint is flexed 90 degrees and the osteotomy is completed by sawing with the wire while keeping the wire perpendicular to the long axis of the antebrachium.

F. The olecranon process with the attached triceps muscles may now be reflected proximally to reveal the entire caudal surface of the joint. If the anconeus muscle is intact, an incision is made through the muscle and the underlying joint capsule near their attachments on the medial condyle; if possible, the branch of the collateral ulnar vessel that penetrates the muscle is preserved.

G. Maximum exposure of the intra-articular area is gained by complete flexion of the joint.

Closure:

No attempt is made to close the incision in the anconeus. A bone screw or threaded Steinman pin is used to secure the tip of the olecranon to the shaft. This screw or pin should be as large as possible, since it is subjected to considerable stress due to the pull of the triceps muscle. The cranial borders of the triceps are sutured to the surrounding deep fascia, and subcutaneous sutures are used to pull the fat and fascia together and to take some of the tension off the skin sutures.

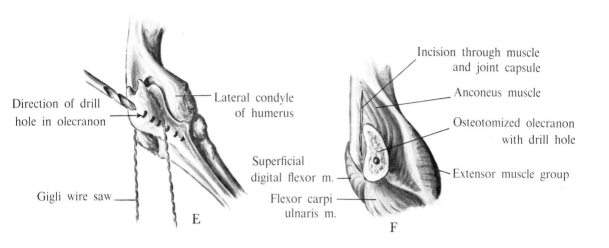

Direction of drill
hole in olecranon

Lateral condyle
of humerus

Incision through muscle
and joint capsule

Anconeus muscle

Osteotomized olecranon
with drill hole

Superficial
digital flexor m.

Extensor muscle group

Gigli wire saw

Flexor carpi
ulnaris m.

E

F

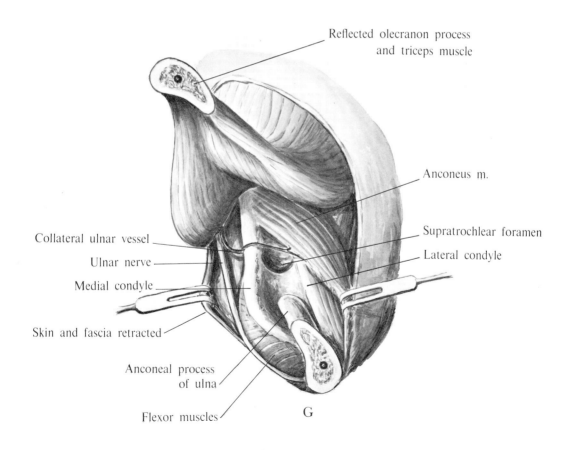

Reflected olecranon process
and triceps muscle

Anconeus m.

Collateral ulnar vessel

Supratrochlear foramen

Ulnar nerve

Lateral condyle

Medial condyle

Skin and fascia retracted

Anconeal process
of ulna

Flexor muscles

G

Page 57

APPROACH TO THE OLECRANON PROCESS AND
PROXIMAL SHAFT OF THE ULNA

INDICATION:

Open reduction of fractures of the olecranon process and proximal shaft of the ulna.

DESCRIPTION OF PROCEDURE:

A. The skin incision commences at the olecranon and follows the prominent caudal border of the ulna distally.

B. Subcutaneous fat and fascia are incised directly under the skin incision and are undermined to allow their retraction with the skin. The deep antebrachial fascia is incised between the extensor carpi ulnaris and the flexor carpi ulnaris.

C. The extensor carpi ulnaris is elevated and retracted laterally by blunt dissection between the muscle and the bone. The flexor carpi ulnaris is elevated subperiosteally to retract it from the bone.

CLOSURE:

Closure of the deep fascial incision will hold the muscles in proper position.

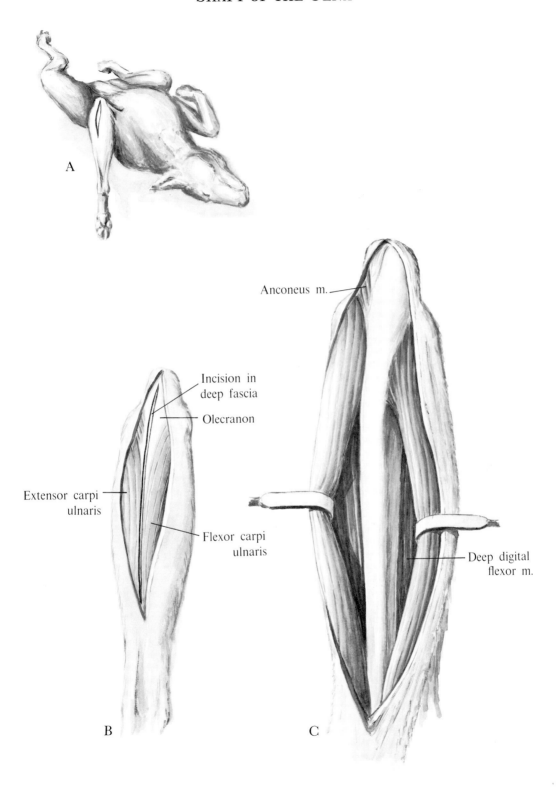

A

Anconeus m.

Incision in
deep fascia

Olecranon

Extensor carpi
ulnaris

Flexor carpi
ulnaris

Deep digital
flexor m.

B

C

APPROACH TO THE DISTAL SHAFT OF THE ULNA

Indications:

1. Osteotomy of the ulna for correction of curvature of the radius.
2. Open reduction of fractures.

Description of Procedure:

A. The skin incision is made directly over the lateral surface of the bone, commencing at its distal end and proceeding proximally half the length of the bone.

B. The incision of the subcutaneous fascia and the retraction of the margins of the skin reveal the tendon of the extensor carpi ulnaris lateral to the bone and the tendon of the lateral digital extensor cranial to the bone.

The deep antebrachial fascia is incised directly over the bone between these two tendons, and the incision is continued through the periosteum.

C. The extensor carpi ulnaris is elevated caudolaterally following subperiosteal elevation, which is made necessary by the firm attachment of the antebrachial fascia to the bone. The lateral digital extensor, the extensor pollicis longus, and the abductor pollicis longus are elevated subperiosteally and retracted cranially to expose the shaft of the bone. The deep digital flexor (ulnar head) muscle lies loosely on the caudal surface of the bone and may be elevated caudally as needed.

Closure:

The deep antebrachial and subcutaneous fasciae are closed in one layer.

PLATE 23. APPROACH TO THE DISTAL SHAFT OF THE ULNA

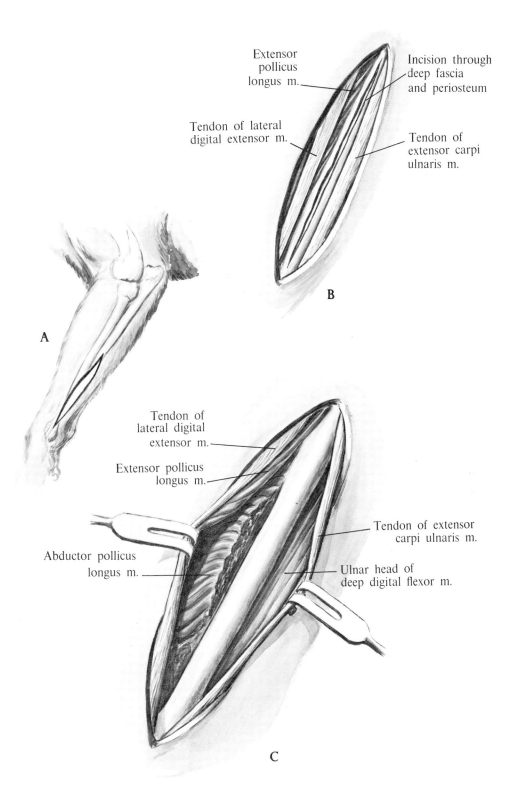

Extensor pollicus longus m.

Incision through deep fascia and periosteum

Tendon of lateral digital extensor m.

Tendon of extensor carpi ulnaris m.

A

B

Tendon of lateral digital extensor m.

Extensor pollicus longus m.

Tendon of extensor carpi ulnaris m.

Abductor pollicus longus m.

Ulnar head of deep digital flexor m.

C

APPROACH TO THE HEAD OF THE RADIUS AND
THE ELBOW JOINT

INDICATIONS:

    1. Open reduction of luxations of the radial head associated with fracture of the radius or ulna.

    2. Ostectomy of the radial head.

DESCRIPTION OF PROCEDURE:

A. The curved incision commences proximal to the lateral humeral epicondyle, crosses the joint, and runs along the lateral surface of the proximal radius. The incision ends at the distal end of the upper fourth of the radius. The subcutaneous fascia is incised on the same line.

B. The skin and subcutaneous fascia are undermined and retracted. The deep antebrachial fascia is incised between the common and lateral digital extensor muscles, and the incision is continued into the intermuscular septum between these muscles. In order to protect the underlying radial nerve, this incision should only be deep enough to allow separation of the muscles.

C. Blunt separation and undermining of the common and lateral digital extensors allows their retraction and the exposure of the underlying supinator muscle. Note the radial nerve emerging from the deep lateral face of the muscle and also the branches of the nerve that terminate in the digital extensor muscles. The nerve must be protected throughout the remainder of the procedure. Although retraction of the nerve is not shown in the accompanying plates, it may be necessary in order to work safely in this area.

An incision is next made through the aponeurosis of the supinator muscle and into the joint capsule. A small stump of muscle should be left on the bone to allow suturing to the belly of the muscle at closure.

D. The supinator is carefully freed from the radius by blunt dissection, with care being taken not to injure the radial nerve. Distal retraction of the muscle will expose the head of the radius.

CLOSURE:

The supinator muscle is sutured to its area of origin by interrupted mattress sutures. The deep fascial incision is closed separately from the subcutaneous fascia.

COMMENTS:

If greater exposure of the joint capsule is required, either or both of the digital extensor muscles are transected near their origins on the lateral epicondyle.

In the *cat*, the radial nerve will be found superficial to the supinator muscle rather than deep as shown in illustration C.

PLATE 24. APPROACH TO THE HEAD OF THE RADIUS AND THE ELBOW JOINT

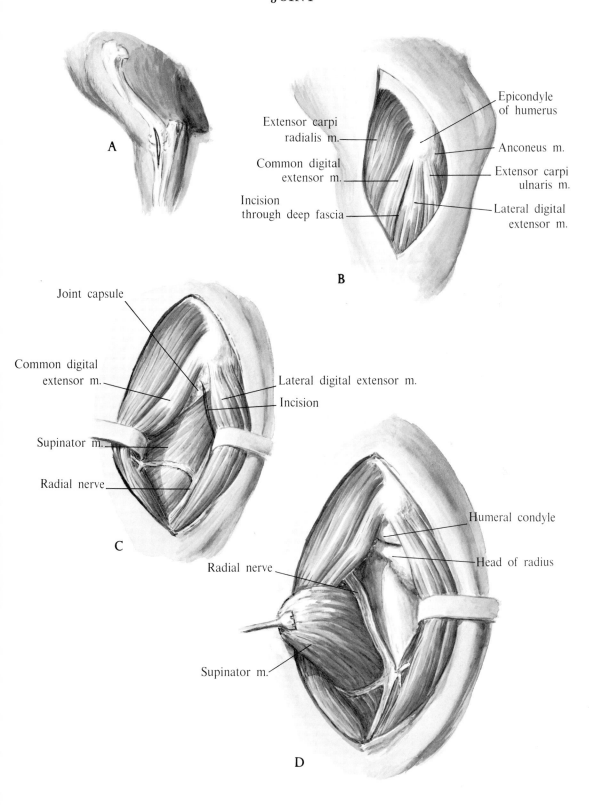

A

Extensor carpi radialis m.

Common digital extensor m.

Incision through deep fascia

Epicondyle of humerus

Anconeus m.

Extensor carpi ulnaris m.

Lateral digital extensor m.

B

Joint capsule

Common digital extensor m.

Supinator m.

Radial nerve

Lateral digital extensor m.

Incision

C

Radial nerve

Supinator m.

Humeral condyle

Head of radius

D

APPROACH TO THE PROXIMAL SHAFT OF THE RADIUS

INDICATION:

Open reduction of fractures in the proximal half of the shaft of the radius.

DESCRIPTION OF PROCEDURE:

A.   The lateral epicondyle of the humerus marks the proximal point of the skin incision, which then crosses the joint and curves cranially to run between the radius and ulna to the midpoint of the radius.

B.   The subcutaneous fat and fascia are incised directly under the skin incision. The fascia is undermined and retracted with the skin to expose the muscles. An incision is made in the deep fascia and is continued into the intermuscular septum between the common and lateral digital extensors. These muscles are easily separated by blunt dissection proximally, but sharp dissection is necessary to separate them distally.

C.   The separation between the common and lateral digital extensors is developed sufficiently to allow retraction of these muscles. The proximal portion of the common extensor must be freed from the radius by blunt dissection in order to allow adequate elevation.

Care must be taken to protect the radial nerve as it emerges from under the supinator muscle.

CLOSURE:

Subcutaneous and deep fasciae are closed in one tier of sutures.

COMMENTS:

Should it be necessary to expose the ulna simultaneously, an incision is made between the lateral digital extensor and the extensor carpi ulnaris. As this separation is developed by blunt dissection, the lateral surface of the ulna is exposed.

PLATE 25. APPROACH TO THE PROXIMAL SHAFT OF THE RADIUS

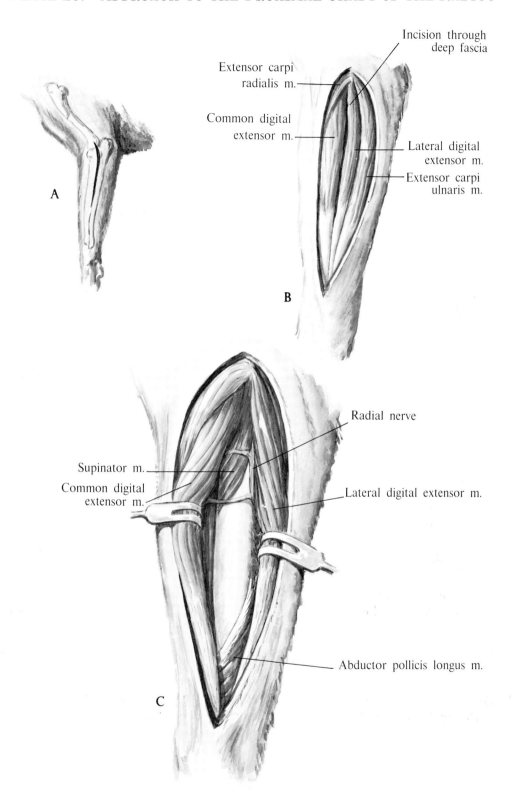

Incision through deep fascia

Extensor carpi radialis m.

Common digital extensor m.

Lateral digital extensor m.

Extensor carpi ulnaris m.

A

B

Radial nerve

Supinator m.

Common digital extensor m.

Lateral digital extensor m.

Abductor pollicis longus m.

C

APPROACH TO THE DISTAL SHAFT OF THE RADIUS

INDICATIONS:

1. Open reduction of fractures.
2. Osteotomy of the radius for correction of angular deformity.

DESCRIPTION OF PROCEDURE:

A. The skin incision is made on the craniomedial aspect of the leg, commencing at the styloid process of the radius and continuing proximally one fourth to one half the length of the bone. The cephalic vein crosses the incision and should be avoided.

B. Subcutaneous fascia is carefully incised in the same line as the skin, and the cephalic vein is undermined and elevated from the bone.

The deep antebrachial and carpal fasciae are now incised directly over the exposed medial surface of the radius. The incision passes under the elevated cephalic vein if the distal end of the bone is to be exposed.

C. Elevation of the extensor carpi radialis is easily accomplished by blunt dissection proximal to the level of the cephalic vein. Distal to this point the tendon of the muscle must be elevated subperiosteally.

The flexor carpi radialis, the deep digital flexor, and the radial artery and vein are elevated as a unit. Some care must be taken to avoid severing the vessels. These muscles and vessels are readily separated from the bone by blunt dissection.

The incision of the fascial intermuscular septum between the pronator teres muscle and the flexors will allow better exposure of the radius in this area.

CLOSURE:

Deep and subcutaneous fasciae may be closed in one layer, but it must be certain that the cephalic vein is not impinged upon by the sutures.

Page 66

PLATE 26. APPROACH TO THE DISTAL SHAFT OF THE RADIUS

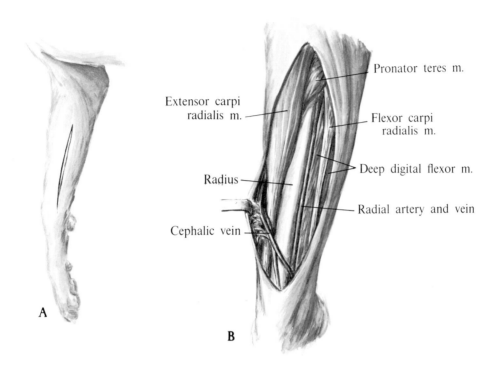

A

B

Pronator teres m.

Extensor carpi
radialis m.

Flexor carpi
radialis m.

Deep digital flexor m.

Radius

Radial artery and vein

Cephalic vein

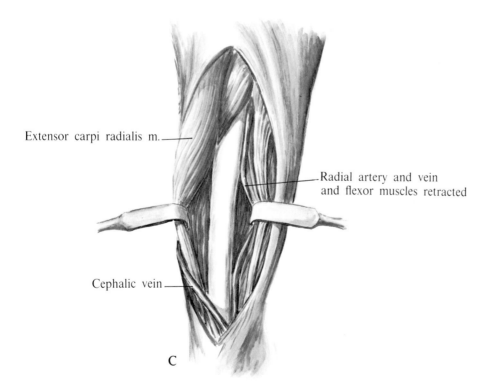

Extensor carpi radialis m.

Radial artery and vein
and flexor muscles retracted

Cephalic vein

C

APPROACH TO THE DISTAL END OF THE RADIUS
AND THE RADIOCARPAL JOINT

INDICATIONS:

1. Open reduction of fractures of the distal radius.
2. Open reduction of luxations of the joint.
3. Arthrodesis of the joint.
4. Removal of loose bodies from the joint.

DESCRIPTION OF PROCEDURE:

A.   The skin incision is made on the mid-dorsal surface of the joint and extends from the juncture of the cephalic and accessory cephalic veins to the middle of the metacarpus. The incision is lateral to the accessory cephalic vein and curves laterally at its distal end to follow the vein.

Subcutaneous fascia is likewise incised just lateral to the vein, enough fascia being left on the vein to allow the placing of sutures in this tissue during closure. The vein and fascia are undermined and retracted medially with the skin.

B.   The deep fascia and the joint capsule are incised midway between the tendon of the extensor carpi radialis and the tendon of the common digital extensor. The limits of this incision are the abductor pollicis longus muscle proximally and the distal border of the radial carpal bone distally. The incision is then deepened to penetrate the periosteum on the distal end of the radius.

C.   The periosteum is elevated medially and laterally to allow the retraction of the tendons without disturbing their sheaths. The fat pad attached to the extensor carpi radialis tendon may be trimmed if necessary to allow visualization of the joint cavity. The styloid process of the ulna may be exposed by continued lateral elevation of the periosteum and retraction of the lateral digital extensor tendon.

CLOSURE:

The area is closed in layers: the joint capsule and deep fascia in one layer, followed by the subcutaneous fascia.

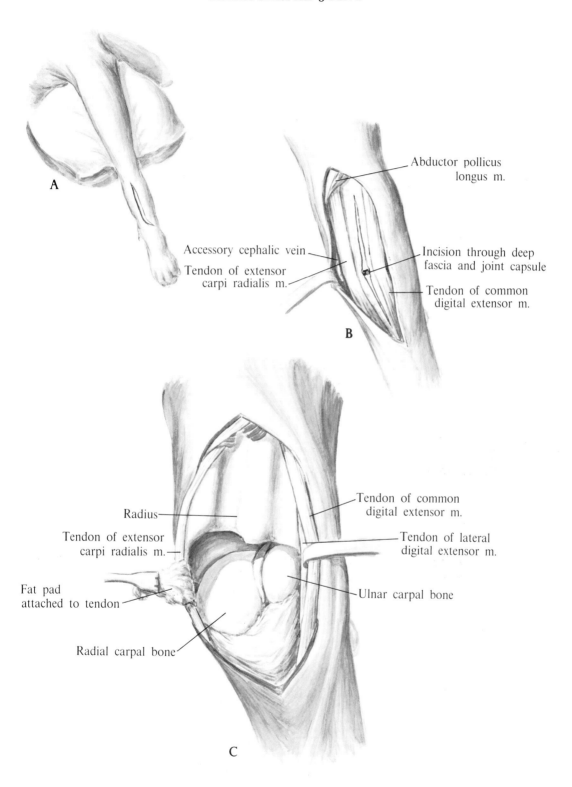

A

Abductor pollicus
longus m.

Accessory cephalic vein

Tendon of extensor
carpi radialis m.

Incision through deep
fascia and joint capsule

Tendon of common
digital extensor m.

B

Radius

Tendon of extensor
carpi radialis m.

Fat pad
attached to tendon

Radial carpal bone

Tendon of common
digital extensor m.

Tendon of lateral
digital extensor m.

Ulnar carpal bone

C

APPROACH TO THE ACCESSORY CARPAL BONE

INDICATION:

Resection of the abductor digiti quinti muscle and removal of bone chips from fractured accessory carpal bone.

DESCRIPTION OF PROCEDURE:

A. The skin incision angles across the lateral surface of the carpus, beginning over the accessory carpal bone and running to the proximal end of metacarpal V. Subcutaneous fascia is incised and retracted with the skin.

B. An incision is made through the deep fascia along the cranial border of the abductor digiti quinti muscle. The incision continues proximally through the palmar carpal transverse ligament, which lies over the accessory carpal bone.

C. Retraction and undermining of the abductor muscle will expose the free end of the accessory carpal bone.

CLOSURE:

Deep and subcutaneous fascia are closed in one layer.

COMMENTS:

Fractures of the accessory carpal, like the central tarsal, occur almost exclusively in track-raced greyhounds, and always in the right carpus.

PLATE 28. APPROACH TO THE ACCESSORY CARPAL BONE

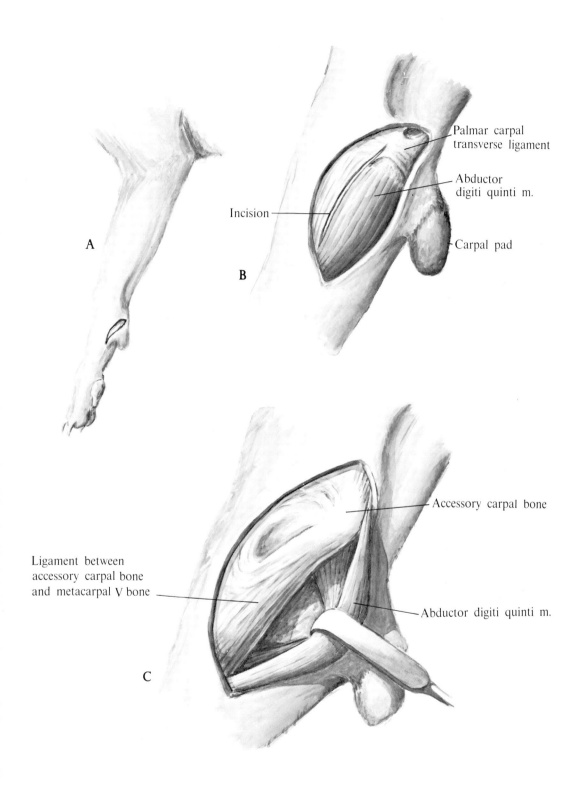

A

B

Incision

Palmar carpal transverse ligament

Abductor digiti quinti m.

Carpal pad

C

Ligament between accessory carpal bone and metacarpal V bone

Accessory carpal bone

Abductor digiti quinti m.

Page 71

APPROACHES TO THE METACARPAL BONES

INDICATION:

Open reduction of fractures.

DESCRIPTION OF PROCEDURE:

The anatomy shown here is considerably simplified compared to that in a live animal. Only the important structures are shown; other elements such as small tendons and blood vessels have been omitted. In an average sized dog these structures are so small as to preclude their identification and preservation during surgery.

The incisional technique varies according to the bone or bones to be exposed. A single bone is approached by an incision directly over the bone, and two adjoining bones by an incision between them. If more than two bones need be exposed, two parallel longitudinal incisions or a single curved incision can be used. The curved incision commences at the proximal end of metacarpal II, runs laterally to the midshaft of metacarpal V, and then curves medially again to end over the distal end of metacarpal II. The crescent-shaped skin flap can be elevated and retracted to expose a large part of all four bones.

To expose metacarpals II and III the deep fascia is incised over bone II, and the vessels and tendons are then undermined and retracted laterally. Deep fascia is incised over bone V to expose bones IV and V. Tendons and vessels are again undermined and retracted medially. Exposure of bone IV sometimes requires an incision between tendons followed by sufficient dissection of the tendons from the surrounding fascia to allow their separation and retraction.

CLOSURE:

Deep fascia is closed to insure that tendons and vessels are securely held in their proper positions.

COMMENTS:

A deep layer of small blood vessels is found on and between the bones. These vessels are too small to avoid in most animals and the resulting hemorrhage must be controlled by tamponade. Use of a tourniquet is very helpful when the operation is done in the regions below the radiocarpal or hock joint. Do not leave the tourniquet in place for more than one hour, and apply a snug bandage for 72 hours postoperatively to control oozing hemorrhage at the operative site.

Page 72

PLATE 29. APPROACHES TO THE METACARPAL BONES

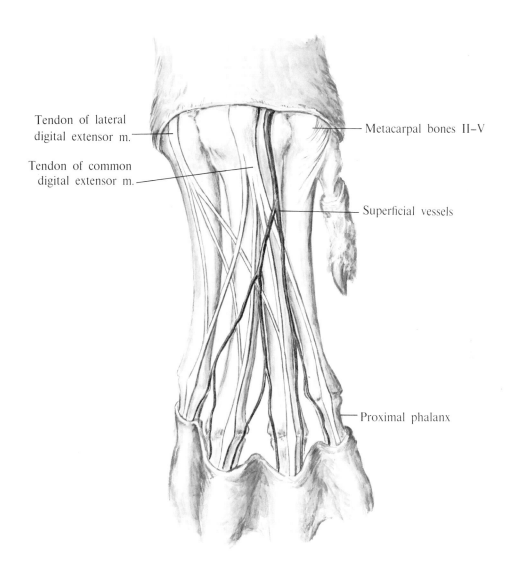

Tendon of lateral
digital extensor m.

Tendon of common
digital extensor m.

Metacarpal bones II–V

Superficial vessels

Proximal phalanx

V | THE PELVIC LIMB

APPROACH TO THE ILIUM THROUGH AN INCISION OVER THE ILIAC CREST

INDICATIONS:

1. Reduction of fractures of the wing and the cranial portion of the body of the ilium.
2. Exposure of donor site for the collection of bone grafts.

DESCRIPTION OF PROCEDURE:

A. The skin incision commences at the crest of the ilium and runs caudally directly over the body of the ilium, terminating approximately above and slightly medial to the greater trochanter. Viewed from above, the incision is approximately parallel to the spine; viewed laterally, the incision slopes ventrally as it progresses toward the ischium.

B. The cutaneus trunci muscle, subcutaneous fat, and deep gluteal fascia are incised in line with the skin incision to expose the middle gluteal muscle and the iliac crest.

C. The middle gluteal muscle is freed from the ilium by the incision of its origin along the crest and dorsal edge of the body of the ilium. This incision is then continued posteriorly in the same line to sever those fibers of the middle gluteal muscle that originate dorsally and medially to the ilium. The superficial gluteal muscle limits the length of this incision posteriorly. The cranial gluteal artery and vein will be found on the surface of the deep gluteal muscle in the deep caudal portion of this incision.

D. The middle gluteal muscle is elevated from the wing of the ilium and retracted laterally. Exposure of the body of the ilium will require the elevation of some of the origin of the deep gluteal muscle.

CLOSURE:

The middle gluteal muscle is sutured back into position by using mattress sutures in the muscle sheath and in the gluteal fascia to pull the muscle back up against the ilium.

COMMENTS:

Elevation of muscle insertions (the iliocostalis and longissimus systems) on the medial surface of the crest and wing allows almost complete exposure of this area of the ilium.

Page 76

PLATE 30. APPROACH TO THE ILIUM THROUGH AN INCISION OVER THE ILIAC CREST

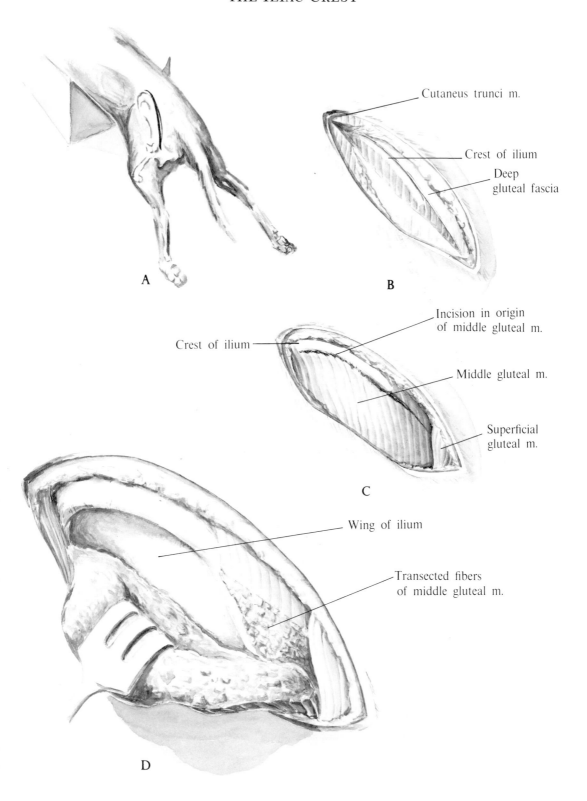

A

Cutaneus trunci m.

Crest of ilium

Deep
gluteal fascia

B

Incision in origin
of middle gluteal m.

Crest of ilium

Middle gluteal m.

Superficial
gluteal m.

C

Wing of ilium

Transected fibers
of middle gluteal m.

D

APPROACH TO THE BODY OF THE ISCHIUM

INDICATION:

Open reduction of fractures of the ischium.

DESCRIPTION OF PROCEDURE:

A.   The sacrotuberous ligament is located by palpation, and the skin incision is made directly over it. The incision extends from the base of the tail to the ischiatic tuberosity. Subcutaneous fat and gluteal fascia are incised on the same line to expose the muscles.

B.   The intermuscular septum between the biceps and the superficial gluteal muscle is incised and the muscles separated. Fat and loose fascia medial to the sacrotuberous ligament are incised and removed or retracted so that the internal obturator muscle is exposed.

C.   The superficial gluteal muscle is undermined and retracted cranially. The sciatic nerve and caudal gluteal artery should now be located and protected. The biceps is partially transected near its origin on the sacrotuberous ligament and the cranial border of the muscle retracted caudally. The internal obturator is transected directly over the body of the ischium.

In the *cat*, the sacrotuberous ligament is not nearly as well developed, being more a condensation of fascia than a distinct structure.

D.   The cut ends of the obturator retract to expose the bone. The sciatic nerve and accompanying vessels are gently dissected free and are retracted with umbilical tape.

CLOSURE:

The transected biceps and obturator muscles are united by horizontal mattress sutures. The gluteal fascia is closed by a suture line, and the often considerable subcutaneous fat by another line.

COMMENTS:

It is not always necessary to transect the biceps as shown here. This step is often valuable, however, in allowing easier retraction of the sciatic nerve and in obtaining more room to manipulate the fractured bone.

Page 78

PLATE 31. APPROACH TO THE BODY OF THE ISCHIUM

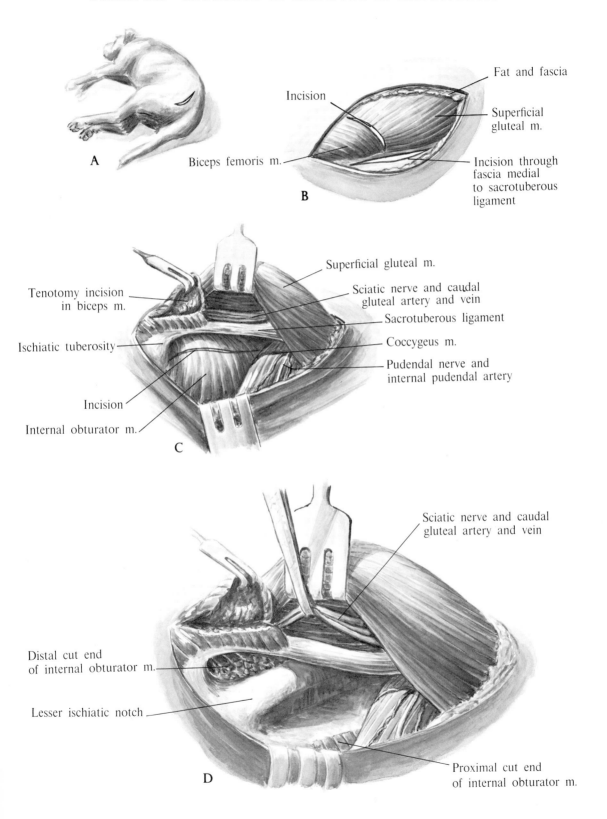

A

Incision

Fat and fascia

Superficial gluteal m.

Biceps femoris m.

Incision through fascia medial to sacrotuberous ligament

B

Tenotomy incision in biceps m.

Superficial gluteal m.

Sciatic nerve and caudal gluteal artery and vein

Sacrotuberous ligament

Ischiatic tuberosity

Coccygeus m.

Pudendal nerve and internal pudendal artery

Incision

Internal obturator m.

C

Sciatic nerve and caudal gluteal artery and vein

Distal cut end of internal obturator m.

Lesser ischiatic notch

Proximal cut end of internal obturator m.

D

Page 79

APPROACH TO THE PUBIS

INDICATIONS:

    1. Open reduction of fractures of the pubis.
    2. Pubic symphysiotomy.

DESCRIPTION OF PROCEDURE:

A.   The skin incision on a male dog is made alongside the penis and extends from the scrotum to a point 1 inch cranial to the pubis. In the female dog and cat the incision is made from the vulva cranially on the midline. The same technique can be applied to the male cat.

B.   The penis is retracted past the midline, following the incision of the fascia alongside the penis and blunt dissection under the organ. A large branch of the external pudendal artery must be ligated to make the fascial incision.

C.   A midline incision commencing just cranial to the pubis is made through the linea alba and continued caudally through the subpelvic tendon to the surface of the pubic symphysis.

D.   The gracilis and adductor muscles are elevated from the pubic symphysis. Avoid opening the peritoneum if possible.

CLOSURE:

The gracilis and adductor muscles are joined at the symphysis by sutures. Care must be taken to insure closure of the peritoneum cranially to the pubis if the peritoneum has been disrupted.

COMMENTS:

Excessive abduction of the hindlegs should be prevented for several days by loosely hobbling the legs together.

PLATE 32. APPROACH TO THE PUBIS

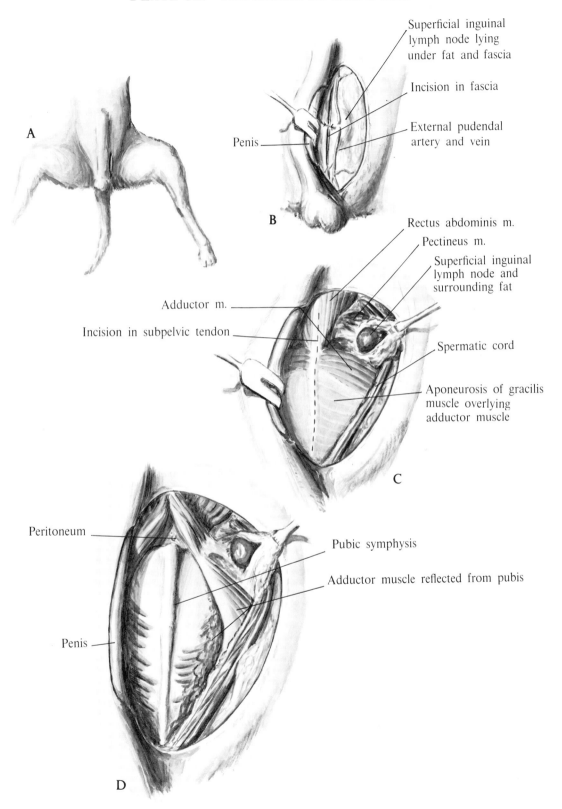

A

B

Superficial inguinal lymph node lying under fat and fascia

Incision in fascia

External pudendal artery and vein

Penis

Rectus abdominis m.

Pectineus m.

Superficial inguinal lymph node and surrounding fat

Adductor m.

Incision in subpelvic tendon

Spermatic cord

Aponeurosis of gracilis muscle overlying adductor muscle

C

Peritoneum

Pubic symphysis

Adductor muscle reflected from pubis

Penis

D

Page 81

APPROACH TO THE ILIUM AND HIP JOINT THROUGH A DORSAL INCISION

INDICATIONS:

1. Reduction of multiple fractures of the ilium.
2. Reduction of fractures of the ilium and concurrent coxofemoral luxations.
3. Reduction of fractures of the ilium and concurrent fractures of the femoral head or neck.

DESCRIPTION OF PROCEDURE:

A. The skin incision, viewed dorsally, is a straight line connecting the iliac crest and the ischiatic tuberosity. When viewed laterally the incision curves ventrally in a halfmoon shape.

B. The incision is developed to bring the gluteal muscles into view by incising the heavy pad of fat and the deep gluteal fascia directly under the skin incision. Care must be taken to avoid severing the sacrotuberous ligament when incising the fascia. The fascia is undermined and widely retracted.

C. The cranial edge of the biceps femoris is reflected caudally over the greater trochanter to expose the insertion of the superficial gluteal muscle. This muscle and the underlying piriformis muscle are then tenotomized close to their insertions. Dorsal retraction of these muscles completely exposes the middle gluteal muscle.

PLATE 33. APPROACH TO THE ILIUM AND HIP JOINT THROUGH A DORSAL INCISION

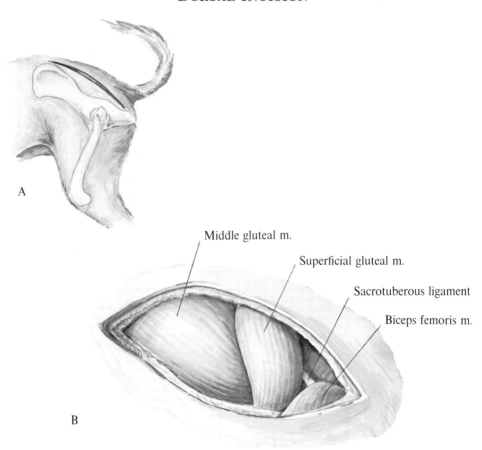

A

Middle gluteal m.

Superficial gluteal m.

Sacrotuberous ligament

Biceps femoris m.

B

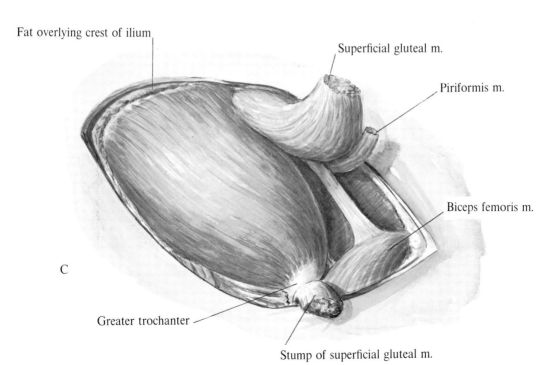

Fat overlying crest of ilium

Superficial gluteal m.

Piriformis m.

Biceps femoris m.

C

Greater trochanter

Stump of superficial gluteal m.

Page 83

D. The middle gluteal muscle is freed from the ilium by incising its fibers of origin along the crest and dorsal edge of the body of the ilium. This incision is then continued caudally in the same line to sever those fibers of the middle gluteal muscle that originate from gluteal fascia dorsally and medially to the ilium. Care should be taken at this point to preserve the cranial gluteal vessels which emerge on the surface of the deep gluteal muscle at the junction of the two bellies of the middle gluteal muscle. The middle gluteal muscle is retracted laterally after it is elevated from its iliac origin.

E. The deep belly of the middle gluteal muscle is tenotomized as close to the greater trochanter as possible, with a small tag of the tendinous insertion being left on the trochanter for reinsertion of the muscle by suturing. Transection should commence from the caudal edge and proceed cranially so as to avoid the sciatic nerve, caudal gluteal vessels, and sacrotuberous ligament. Maximal elevation and retraction of this muscle reveal the dorsal edge of the body of the ilium. Elevation of the sciatic and caudal gluteal vessels allows exposure of a small area of the ischium immediately caudal to the acetabulum.

F. The deep gluteal muscle is undermined close to the trochanter and is divided in a manner similar to that used in dividing the deep belly of the middle gluteal. Careful elevation of the muscle provides exposure of the superior rim of the acetabulum and the lateral surface of the body of the ilium. If further exposure is necessary, part of the origin of the muscle may be elevated subperiosteally from the ilium.

CLOSURE:

Muscles are sutured back in position with interrupted mattress stitches and nonabsorbable suture material. The deep gluteal fascia and fat are closed in separate layers.

D

Periosteal incision

Deep belly of middle gluteal m.

Sciatic n.

Middle gluteal m.

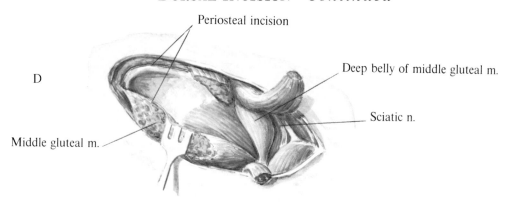

E

Cranial gluteal vessels

Deep belly of middle gluteal m.

Sciatic nerve

Caudal gluteal vessels

Biceps femoris m.

Deep gluteal m.

Stump of deep belly of
middle gluteal m.

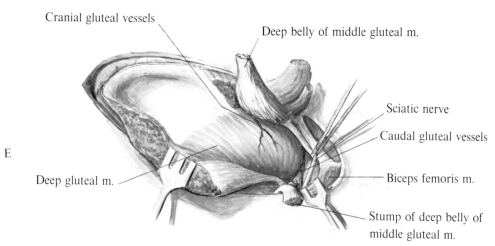

F

Deep gluteal m.

Acetabulum
Joint capsule
incised

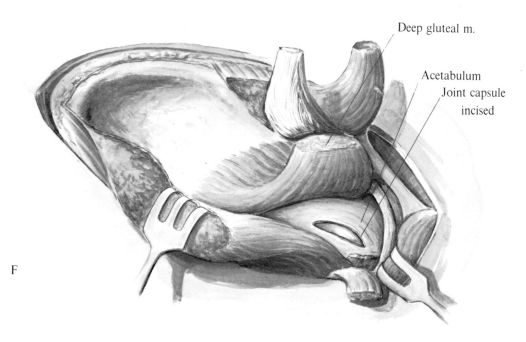

APPROACH TO THE HIP JOINT THROUGH A CRANIOLATERAL INCISION

INDICATIONS:

1. Femoral head ostectomy.
2. Open reduction of fractures of the femoral head and neck.
3. Open reduction of coxofemoral luxations.

DESCRIPTION OF PROCEDURE:

A. The skin incision is centered at the level of the greater trochanter and lies over the cranial border of the shaft of the femur. Distally it extends one third to one half the length of the femur, and proximally it curves cranially to end just short of the dorsal midline.

B. The skin margins are undermined and retracted. An incision is made through the fascia lata and the insertion of the tensor fascia lata muscle along the cranial border of the biceps femoris muscle. It is continued proximally through the gluteal fascia along the cranial border of the superficial gluteal muscle.

C. The fascia lata and the attached tensor fascia lata muscle are retracted cranially and the biceps caudally. Blunt dissection and separation along the neck of the femur with the finger tip allows visualization of a triangle bounded dorsally by the middle and deep gluteal muscles, laterally by the vastus lateralis muscle, and medially by the rectus femoris muscle.

D. Lateral retraction of the combined bellies of the vastus lateralis and intermedius muscles is followed by further blunt dissection to expose the area of the joint. The cranial femoral vessels and the femoral nerve should be protected and preserved if possible. The joint capsule is well covered by loose fatty tissue, which must be cleared away.

E. In most cases exposure is extended if a portion of the insertion of the deep gluteal is transected near its insertion on the trochanter. This allows adequate dorsal retraction of the cranial border of the muscle. Cranial retraction of the rectus femoris muscle further enlarges the exposed area.

   Exposure of the femoral neck is gained by blunt dissection around the bone to allow elevation of the surrounding muscle.

CLOSURE:

One or two sutures are placed in the deep gluteal muscle incision, and the fascia lata and the tensor fascia lata muscle are sutured to the biceps in one layer.

PLATE 35. APPROACH TO THE HIP JOINT THROUGH A CRANIOLATERAL INCISION

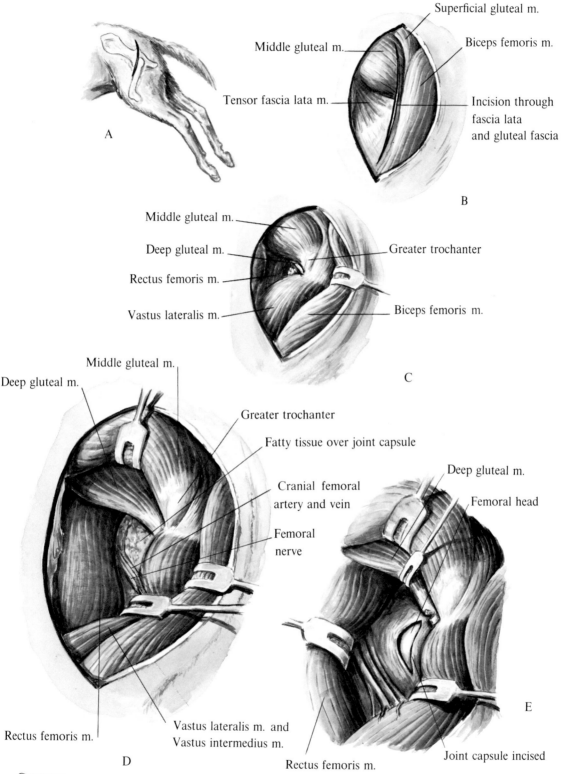

Superficial gluteal m.

Middle gluteal m.

Biceps femoris m.

Tensor fascia lata m.

Incision through fascia lata and gluteal fascia

A

B

Middle gluteal m.

Deep gluteal m.

Rectus femoris m.

Vastus lateralis m.

Greater trochanter

Biceps femoris m.

C

Middle gluteal m.

Deep gluteal m.

Greater trochanter

Fatty tissue over joint capsule

Deep gluteal m.

Femoral head

Cranial femoral artery and vein

Femoral nerve

Rectus femoris m.

Vastus lateralis m. and Vastus intermedius m.

Rectus femoris m.

Joint capsule incised

D

E

COMMENTS:

Exposure of the femoral head is quite limited in the large or very obese dog. This approach is preferred for femoral head ostectomy in all other cases however.

APPROACH TO THE HIP JOINT BY SEPARATION
OF THE GLUTEAL MUSCLE FIBERS

INDICATIONS:

1. Open reduction of coxofemoral luxations.
2. Open reduction of fractures in the area of the acetabulum.

DESCRIPTION OF PROCEDURE:

A. The skin incision extends from the greater trochanter in a cranially curving direction and ends slightly lateral to the dorsal midline.

B. The incision is carried through the subcutaneous fat and gluteal fascia to allow visualization of the superficial and middle gluteal muscles.

C. The fibers of the superficial gluteal muscle are separated by starting at a point directly over the greater trochanter and continuing proximally in the direction of the fibers. Retraction of each half of the superficial gluteal muscle will reveal the underlying middle gluteal muscle.

D. The fibers of the middle gluteal muscle are divided longitudinally by starting at the trochanter and proceeding proximally. When these fibers are completely separated and retracted, the deep belly of the middle gluteal muscle and the underlying deep gluteal muscle are visible. The sciatic nerve and caudal gluteal vessels should be identified at this point, and measures should be taken to protect them.

E. The deep belly of the middle gluteal muscle is best retracted caudally, or alternatively, tenotomized near its insertion on the greater trochanter and retracted cranially. The separation of the fibers of the deep gluteal muscle will expose the shaft of the ilium, the superior rim of the acetabulum, and the joint capsule.

CLOSURE:

Suturing of the gluteal muscles is not necessary. The deep belly of the middle gluteal muscle should be reattached to the greater trochanter if it was tenotomized. The gluteal fascia and fat are closed separately.

COMMENTS:

Although the femoral head and acetabulum can be visualized by this approach, it does not allow much working area for the surgeon.

PLATE 36. APPROACH TO THE HIP JOINT BY SEPARATION OF THE GLUTEAL MUSCLE FIBERS

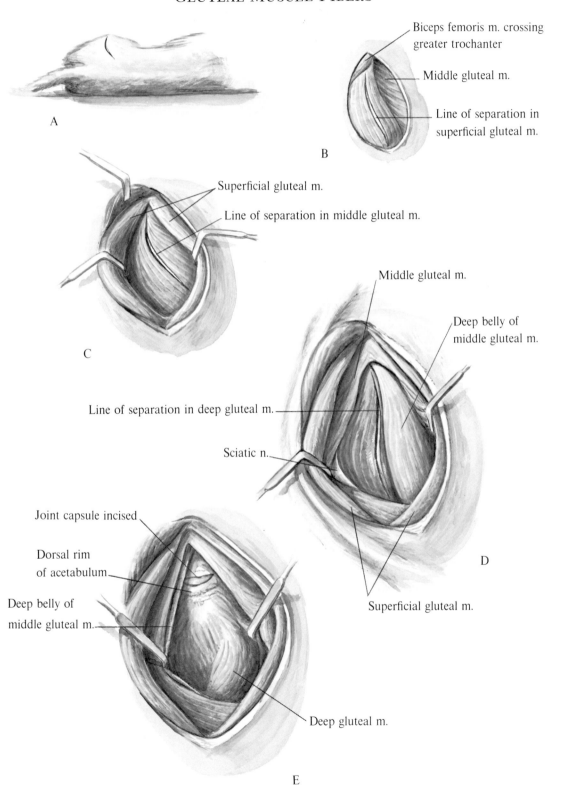

A

Biceps femoris m. crossing greater trochanter

Middle gluteal m.

Line of separation in superficial gluteal m.

B

Superficial gluteal m.

Line of separation in middle gluteal m.

C

Middle gluteal m.

Deep belly of middle gluteal m.

Line of separation in deep gluteal m.

Sciatic n.

Superficial gluteal m.

D

Joint capsule incised

Dorsal rim of acetabulum

Deep belly of middle gluteal m.

Deep gluteal m.

E

Page 89

APPROACH TO THE HIP JOINT AND BODY OF THE ILIUM BY TENOTOMY OF THE GLUTEAL MUSCLES

INDICATIONS:

1. Open reduction of fractures of the femoral head and neck.
2. Open reduction of fractures of the pelvis near the acetabulum.
3. Open reduction of coxofemoral luxations.
4. Installation of femoral head and hip joint prostheses.
5. Femoral head ostectomy and other arthroplastic procedures.

DESCRIPTION OF PROCEDURE:

A. The skin incision follows the craniolateral surface of the femur starting at a point half way down the shaft, extending proximally past the trochanter, and then curving cranially almost to the midline.

B. The fascia lata is incised along the cranial edge of the biceps femoris muscle by starting distally and continuing proximally as far as the skin incision allows.

C. The biceps is reflected caudally and the skin and fascia lata cranially to expose the superficial gluteal muscle and the tensor fascia lata muscle. The tensor fascia lata muscle is transected near its insertion in the trochanter area. The sciatic nerve should be identified as it emerges from under the caudal edge of the middle gluteal muscle, crosses obliquely over the caudal rim of the acetabulum, and continues distally caudal to the neck of the femur. This nerve must be protected throughout the approach.

The borders of the superficial gluteal muscle are developed by dissection from the surrounding fascia, and the muscle is tenotomized in the middle of its tendinous insertion, approximately over the most lateral prominence of the greater trochanter.

D. The superficial gluteal muscle is retracted proximally to expose the middle gluteal muscle, and the belly of this muscle is then undermined near its insertion on the trochanter. The tendinous insertion of the muscle is transected near the trochanter so that some tendinous tissue is retained on both sides of the incision.

E. The free gluteal muscles are retracted dorsally out of the field.

The deep gluteal muscle is then undermined in the same manner as the middle gluteal muscle. (The attachment of the deep gluteal muscle is situated more cranially on the trochanter than the middle gluteal muscle.) The tenotomy is done in the same manner as that described for the middle gluteal.

Page 90

PLATE 37.   APPROACH TO THE HIP JOINT AND BODY OF THE ILIUM BY TENOTOMY OF THE GLUTEAL MUSCLES

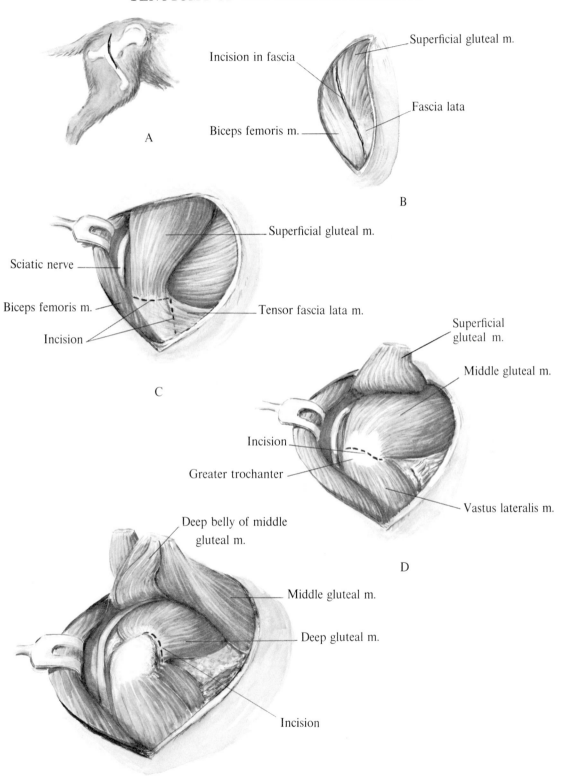

Incision in fascia

Superficial gluteal m.

Fascia lata

Biceps femoris m.

A

B

Sciatic nerve

Biceps femoris m.

Incision

Superficial gluteal m.

Tensor fascia lata m.

C

Superficial gluteal m.

Middle gluteal m.

Incision

Greater trochanter

Vastus lateralis m.

D

Deep belly of middle gluteal m.

Middle gluteal m.

Deep gluteal m.

Incision

E

Page 91

F. The deep gluteal muscle is undermined and retracted proximally. This muscle is tightly adherent to the joint capsule in some cases and is therefore difficult to elevate. The joint capsule and the capsularis muscle are incised half way between the rim of the acetabulum and the insertion of the joint capsule on the femoral neck. This incision is carried cranially around the joint as far as necessary to expose the head of the femur.

G. To expose the shaft of the ilium, the deep gluteal muscle is elevated subperiosteally from the body of the ilium as far cranially as necessary.

Elevation of the sciatic nerve and gemellus muscle will expose a limited area of the shaft of the ischium. The gemellus may be tenotomized near its insertion on the trochanter if necessary.

CLOSURE:

The gluteal muscles are sutured to their insertions by using interrupted mattress sutures of nonabsorbable material. The tensor fascia lata muscle and the fascia lata are closed in one layer.

COMMENTS:

An alternative method of tenotomizing the middle and deep gluteal muscles involves dividing the muscles flush with the trochanter. They are reattached to the bone by means of sutures passed through holes drilled in the trochanter.

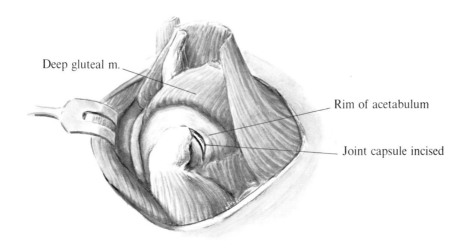

Deep gluteal m.

Rim of acetabulum

Joint capsule incised

F

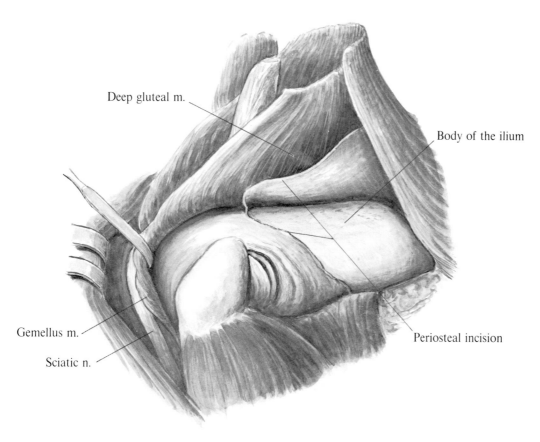

Deep gluteal m.

Body of the ilium

Gemellus m.

Sciatic n.

Periosteal incision

G

Page 93

APPROACH TO THE HIP JOINT AND BODY OF THE ILIUM BY OSTEOTOMY OF THE GREATER TROCHANTER

INDICATIONS:

    1. Open reduction of fractures of the femoral head and neck.
    2. Open reduction of fractures of the pelvis near the acetabulum.
    3. Open reduction of coxofemoral luxations.
    4. Installation of femoral head and hip joint prostheses.
    5. Femoral head ostectomy and other arthroplastic procedures.

EXPLANATORY NOTE:

The procedure is initiated as shown in illustrations A, B, and C of Plate 37, Approach to the Hip Joint and Body of the Ilium by Tenotomy of the Gluteal Muscles (p. 91).

DESCRIPTION OF PROCEDURE:

A. Following the reflection of the superficial gluteal muscle, the middle and deep gluteal muscles are undermined and the trochanter is cut with an osteotome to include the entire insertion of the middle gluteal muscle and as much of the insertion of the deep gluteal muscle as possible.

B. Much of the deep gluteal muscle insertion will be intact following the transection of the trochanter and it should then be cut as shown in illustration E of Plate 37.

CLOSURE:

The trochanter is secured to the shaft by 2 or 3 strands of 26 gauge stainless steel wire passed through holes drilled in the trochanter and in the shaft just below the line of division. The deep and superficial gluteal muscles are sutured to their insertions.

COMMENTS:

Some care should be taken to place the osteotome on the trochanter at an angle to the femoral shaft which corresponds with the angle of the femoral neck relative to the femoral shaft. This makes the line of osteotomy parallel to the dorsal surface of the neck and prevents cutting into the neck. An alternative method of removing the trochanter is by use of a Gigli wire saw, the wire being passed under the gluteal muscles at their attachments on the trochanter.

Page 94

PLATE 39. APPROACH TO THE HIP JOINT AND BODY OF THE ILIUM BY OSTEOTOMY OF THE GREATER TROCHANTER

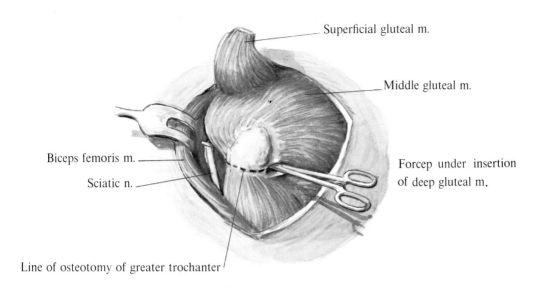

Superficial gluteal m.

Middle gluteal m.

Biceps femoris m.

Sciatic n.

Forcep under insertion of deep gluteal m.

Line of osteotomy of greater trochanter

A

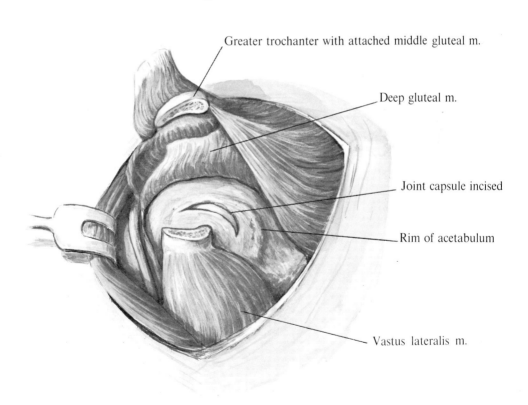

Greater trochanter with attached middle gluteal m.

Deep gluteal m.

Joint capsule incised

Rim of acetabulum

Vastus lateralis m.

B

Page 95

APPROACH TO THE HIP JOINT THROUGH A CAUDOLATERAL INCISION

INDICATIONS:

1. Femoral head ostectomy and other arthroplastic procedures.
2. Open reduction of fractures of the ischium near the acetabulum.
3. Open reduction of coxofemoral luxations.

DESCRIPTION OF PROCEDURE:

A. The curved incision is centered on the caudal surface of the greater trochanter. It starts at a point half way between the dorsal midline and the trochanter and extends through the proximal fourth of the femur.

B. The subcutaneous fat is undermined and retracted with the skin. The fascia lata is incised along the cranial border of the biceps. This incision is approximately as long as the skin incision.

C. The fascia lata is undermined and retracted cranially and the biceps retracted caudally. The sciatic nerve should be visualized at this time and protected throughout the remainder of the procedure.

The area between the sciatic nerve and the neck of the femur is cleared of fat and areolar tissue so that the underlying muscles are visible.

D. With the leg abducted, the gluteal muscles are retracted cranially and lifted to give maximum exposure of the joint capsule. The tendon of the internal obturator and the gemellus are undermined preparatory to being transected.

E. Division of the obturator tendon and the gemellus is accomplished close to their insertions on the femur, but with enough of the insertion being left to allow suturing.

The joint capsule and caudal rim of the acetabulum are now visible. Maximum exposure of the femoral head and neck is attained by inward rotation of the stifle joint.

CLOSURE:

The obturator tendon and gemellus are reattached with mattress sutures. The fascia lata is sutured to the cranial border of the biceps, but the subcutaneous fat and fascia are usually deep enough to require a separate suture line.

COMMENTS:

Except in large dogs, this approach does not give much room in which to work. When used in the open reduction of a craniodorsal coxofemoral luxation, the approach has the merit of good exposure of the acetabulum so that it can be cleaned out before reduction is attempted.

PLATE 40. APPROACH TO THE HIP JOINT THROUGH A CAUDOLATERAL INCISION

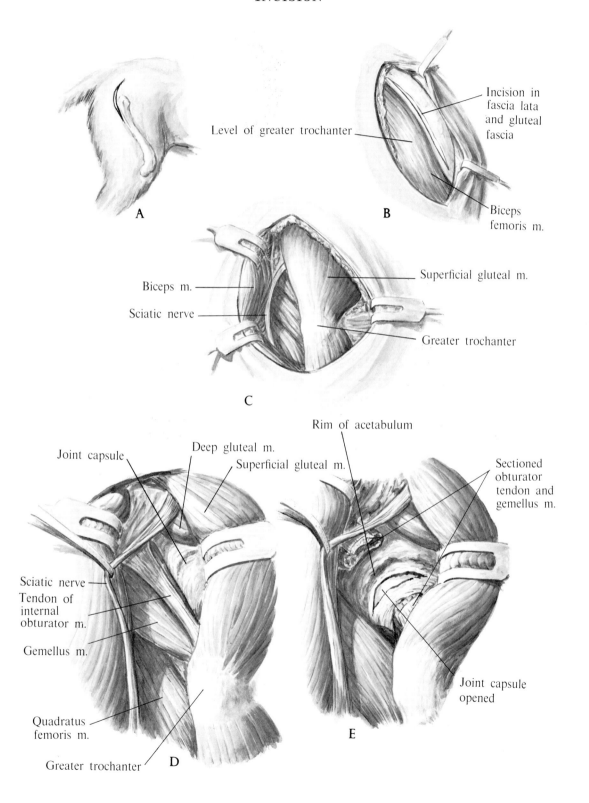

Level of greater trochanter

Incision in fascia lata and gluteal fascia

Biceps femoris m.

A

B

Biceps m.

Sciatic nerve

Superficial gluteal m.

Greater trochanter

C

Rim of acetabulum

Joint capsule

Deep gluteal m.

Superficial gluteal m.

Sectioned obturator tendon and gemellus m.

Sciatic nerve

Tendon of internal obturator m.

Gemellus m.

Quadratus femoris m.

Greater trochanter

Joint capsule opened

D

E

Page 97

APPROACH TO THE HIP JOINT THROUGH A VENTRAL INCISION

INDICATIONS:

    1. Open reduction of ventral luxations of the femoral head.
    2. Open reduction of fractures of the ventral rim of the acetabulum.
    3. Ostectomy of the femoral head.

DESCRIPTION OF PROCEDURE:

A. The skin incision is made in the form of a **T**. The cord-like pectineus muscle is palpated with the hip in extreme abduction. One leg of the incision runs in the fold of the groin and crosses the origin of the pectineus. This incision terminates caudally at the base of the scrotum or at the vulva. The second incision runs directly along the pectineus for a distance of one fourth to one third the length of the femur.

B. The fascia is opened in line with the skin incision and the skin flaps undermined and retracted. The belly of the pectineus muscle is mobilized by blunt dissection, with care being taken to protect the femoral artery, vein, and nerve which run along the cranial border of the muscle. The pectineus is transected at its midpoint by a step-like incision.

PLATE 41. APPROACH TO THE HIP JOINT THROUGH A VENTRAL INCISION

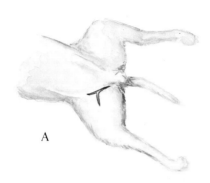

A

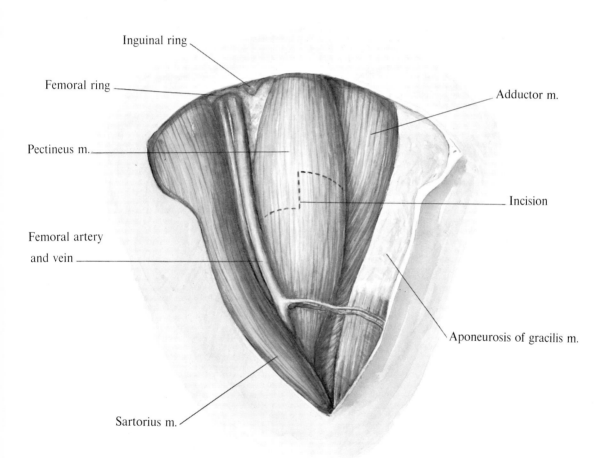

Inguinal ring

Femoral ring

Adductor m.

Pectineus m.

Incision

Femoral artery
and vein

Aponeurosis of gracilis m.

Sartorius m.

B

APPROACH TO THE HIP JOINT THROUGH A VENTRAL
INCISION—*Continued*

C. The pectineus muscle is reflected to reveal the iliopsoas muscle and the deep femoral artery and vein which runs caudally and medial to the acetabular portion of the pelvis. It may be necessary to free these vessels from the surrounding fascia and to retract them proximally.

The iliopsoas muscle lies oblique to the femoral shaft and runs in a craniodorsal direction under the femoral and deep femoral vessels.

D. An interval between the iliopsoas and the adductor muscles is developed by blunt dissection. Retraction of the iliopsoas cranially and the adductor caudally exposes the rim of the acetabulum. The joint capsule is shown incised so as to reveal the femoral head. Greater exposure of the neck of the femur can be developed by further separation and retraction of the iliopsoas and adductor muscles.

CLOSURE:

The cut edges of the belly of the pectineus are apposed by interrupted horizontal mattress sutures placed in the muscle sheath around the entire circumference of the muscle. The sutures are started on the deep surface of the muscle and are placed before apposing the cut surfaces. The suture line is continued on the superficial surface to complete the closure of the pectineus.

COMMENTS:

Exposure of the joint by this approach is quite limited, and its use is therefore quite limited.

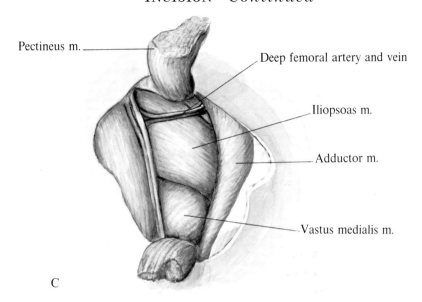

Pectineus m.

Deep femoral artery and vein

Iliopsoas m.

Adductor m.

Vastus medialis m.

C

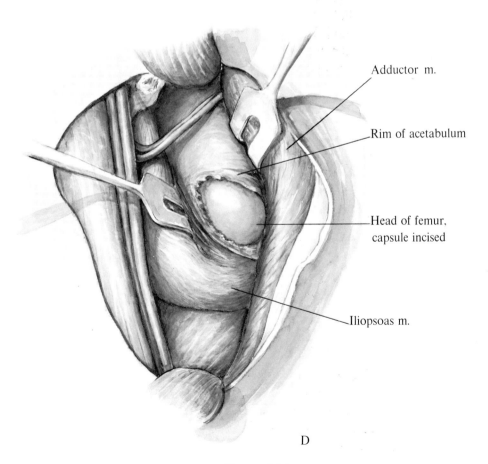

Adductor m.

Rim of acetabulum

Head of femur, capsule incised

Iliopsoas m.

D

Page 101

APPROACH TO THE TROCHANTERIC PORTION
OF THE FEMUR

INDICATION:

Open reduction of fractures in the trochanteric and subtrochanteric portions of the femur.

DESCRIPTION OF PROCEDURE:

A. The skin incision curves from a point dorsal and cranial to the trochanter, extends over the lateral surface of the trochanter, and ends distally a fourth of the way down the shaft of the femur.

B. The subcutaneous fat and fascia are incised and cleared from the area so that the fascia lata can be clearly visualized. An incision is made through the fascia lata along the cranial border of the biceps femoris muscle.

C. The biceps is reflected caudally and the skin and fascia lata cranially. The borders of the superficial gluteal muscle are developed by dissection from the surrounding fascia, and the tendon of insertion of this muscle is cut near its insertion on the femur. Sufficient stump is left distally to allow suturing to the belly of the muscle at closure.

D. The stumps of the superficial gluteal muscle are retracted proximally and distally to expose the greater trochanter and the middle gluteal muscle. An incision is now made through the fibers of origin of the vastus lateralis muscle along the ridge of the third trochanter of the femur. This incision is deepened to include the periosteum.

E. Subperiosteal elevation of this proximal lateral portion of the vastus lateralis and the insertion of the superficial gluteal muscle exposes the shaft of the femur. The adductor muscle on the caudal side of the bone can also be elevated from the bone to give additional exposure.

CLOSURE:

The vastus lateralis muscle is reattached to the periosteum by sutures. This may require the elevation of the periosteum on the proximal side of the incision for a sufficient distance to allow sutures to be placed in it. Interrupted mattress sutures are used in the tendon of the superficial gluteal muscle. The fascia lata is then sutured to the biceps femoris.

Page 102

PLATE 43. APPROACH TO THE TROCHANTERIC PORTION OF THE FEMUR

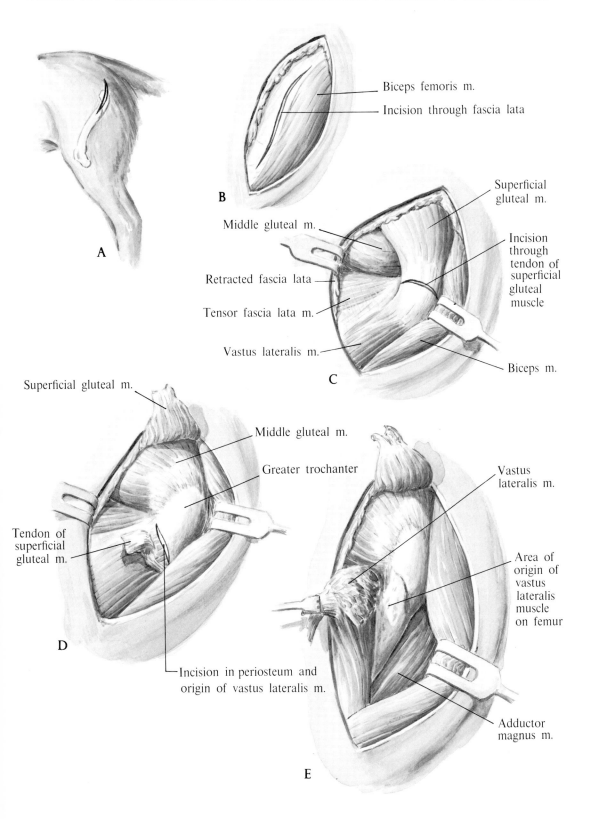

A

B
— Biceps femoris m.
— Incision through fascia lata

C
Middle gluteal m.
Retracted fascia lata —
Tensor fascia lata m. —
Vastus lateralis m. —
Superficial gluteal m.
Incision through tendon of superficial gluteal muscle
Biceps m.

D
Superficial gluteal m.
Middle gluteal m.
Greater trochanter
Tendon of superficial gluteal m.
Incision in periosteum and origin of vastus lateralis m.

E
Vastus lateralis m.
Area of origin of vastus lateralis muscle on femur
Adductor magnus m.

Page 103

APPROACH TO THE SHAFT OF THE FEMUR

INDICATION:

Open reduction of fractures of the shaft proximal to the supracondylar area.

DESCRIPTION OF PROCEDURE:

A. The skin incision is made along the craniolateral border of the shaft of the bone from the level of the greater trochanter to the level of the patella. The subcutaneous fat and superficial fascia are incised directly under the skin incision.

B. The skin margins are undermined and retracted. The fascia lata is incised along the cranial border of the biceps femoris muscle. This incision extends the entire length of the skin incision.

C. Caudal retraction of the biceps and cranial retraction of the vastus lateralis muscle reveal the shaft of the femur. It is necessary to incise the fascial intermuscular septum between these muscles on the lateral shaft of the bone in order to adequately retract the vastus lateralis.

D. The adductor muscle, which inserts on the caudal aspect of the shaft of the femur, may be subperiosteally reflected if necessary. The vastus intermedius muscle on the cranial surface of the shaft is retracted by freeing the loose fascia between the muscle and the bone.

CLOSURE:

Closure consists of suturing the fascia lata to the cranial border of the biceps muscle in one tier and the subcutaneous fat and fascia in a second tier.

PLATE 44. APPROACH TO THE SHAFT OF THE FEMUR

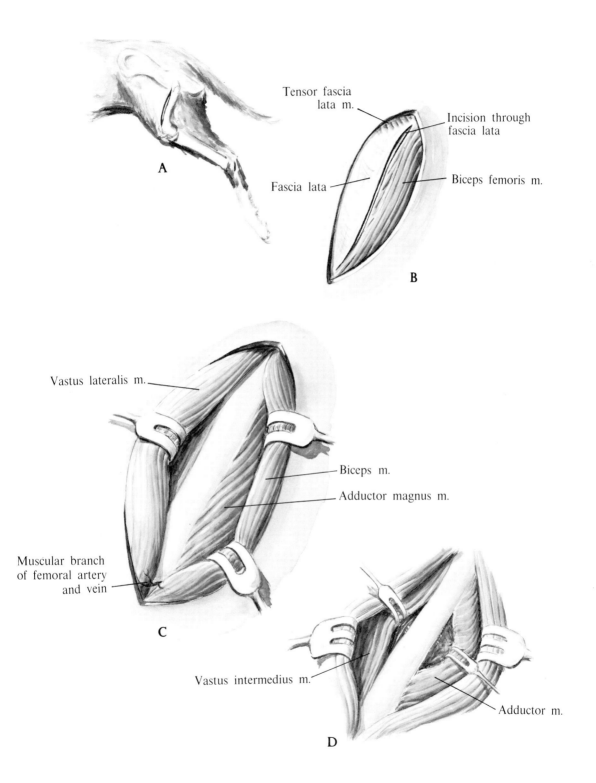

A

Tensor fascia
lata m.

Incision through
fascia lata

Fascia lata

Biceps femoris m.

B

Vastus lateralis m.

Biceps m.

Adductor magnus m.

Muscular branch
of femoral artery
and vein

C

Vastus intermedius m.

Adductor m.

D

APPROACH TO THE DISTAL END OF THE FEMUR AND THE STIFLE JOINT THROUGH A LATERAL INCISION

INDICATIONS:

1. Open reduction of supracondylar, intracondylar, and distal epiphyseal fractures of the femur.
2. Exploration of the stifle joint.
3. Removal of the lateral meniscus.
4. Removal of loose bodies from the cranial compartment of the stifle joint.

DESCRIPTION OF PROCEDURES:

A. After palpation of the patella and lateral trochlear ridge, a curved parapatellar skin incision is made extending from the distal fourth of the femur over the trochlear ridge to the tibial tuberosity. The subcutaneous fascia is incised in the same line as the skin incision. The fascia lata and lateral fascia of the stifle joint are exposed by undermining the subcutaneous fat and fascia, which are then retracted with the skin.

B. Another curved incision, similar to that in the skin, is made through the fascia lata along the cranial border of the biceps. The incision continues distally into the lateral fascia of the stifle joint. As it crosses the trochlear ridge it curves to parallel the lateral border of the patella and the patellar tendon. Enough fascia is left on the lateral edge of the patella to receive sutures when the joint is closed.

C. The biceps and attached lateral joint fascia are elevated and retracted caudally. In separating the biceps from the vastus lateralis, an intermuscular septum formed from the fascia lata is found attached to the femur. This fascia must be trimmed free to allow mobilization of the vastus lateralis and biceps. A parapatellar incision is now made through the joint capsule.

D. With the joint extended, the patella and vastus lateralis can be luxated medially. Lateral retraction of the joint capsule with the biceps and lateral joint fascia fully exposes the interior of the joint.

CLOSURE:

The joint capsule and lateral fascia of the stifle joint are closed in one layer with nonabsorbable suture material. A Lembert pattern is used to prevent any suture material from penetrating the joint capsule. The fascia lata incision must also be sutured.

COMMENTS:

This approach is preferred over the medial approach (Plate 46, p. 109) for the reduction of supracondylar and epiphyseal fractures because it affords superior exposure and ease of retrograde insertion of intramedullary pins.

PLATE 45. APPROACH TO THE DISTAL END OF THE FEMUR AND THE STIFLE JOINT THROUGH A LATERAL INCISION

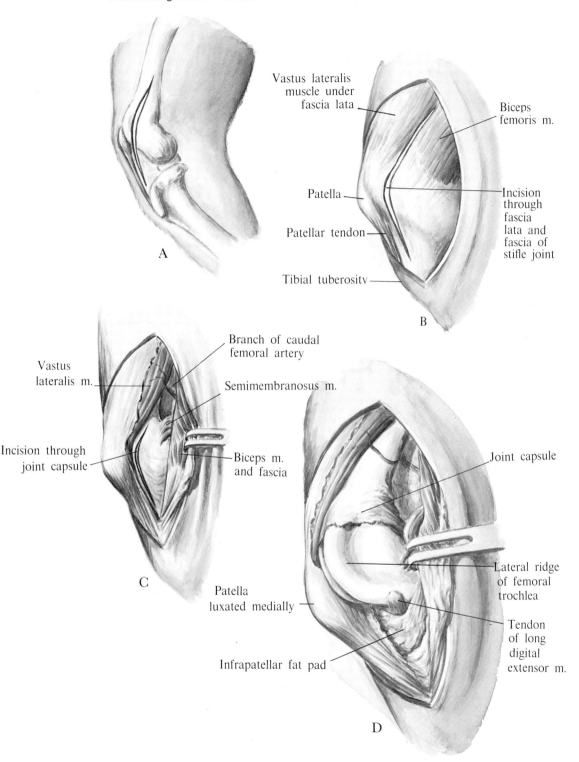

Vastus lateralis muscle under fascia lata

Biceps femoris m.

Patella

Patellar tendon

Incision through fascia lata and fascia of stifle joint

Tibial tuberosity

A

B

Vastus lateralis m.

Branch of caudal femoral artery

Semimembranosus m.

Incision through joint capsule

Biceps m. and fascia

Joint capsule

C

Patella luxated medially

Lateral ridge of femoral trochlea

Tendon of long digital extensor m.

Infrapatellar fat pad

D

By combining this approach with the Approach to the Shaft of the Femur (Plate 44, p. 105), the entire bone can be exposed. It should be noted that the joint capsule usually need not be incised to expose supracondylar fractures, but it is always incised when the fracture is at the epiphyseal line, which is intracapsular.

APPROACH TO THE DISTAL END OF THE FEMUR AND THE STIFLE JOINT THROUGH A MEDIAL INCISION

INDICATIONS:

1. Open reduction of supracondylar, intracondylar, and distal epiphyseal fractures of the femur.
2. Exploration of the stifle joint.
3. Removal of the medial meniscus.
4. Removal of loose bodies in the cranial compartment of the stifle joint.

DESCRIPTION OF PROCEDURE:

A. The skin incision is parallel and medial to the cranial midline of the leg and extends over the distal fourth of the femur to the level of the tibial tuberosity.

The subcutaneous fascia is incised in the same line to expose the medial fascia of the stifle joint.

B. The cranial skin flap and subcutaneous fascia are undermined and retracted laterally past the midline to expose the patella and the patellar tendon.

A parapatellar incision through the medial fascia of the stifle joint is started at the level of the tibia and continued proximally into the sartorius muscle. This incision must leave enough fascia on the medial edge of the patella to allow sutures to be placed in it.

C. This incision is deepened to include the joint capsule and is continued proximally past the capsule into the vastus medialis muscle, which is split in the direction of its fibers.

D. The patella is luxated laterally and the stifle joint flexed to allow examination of the joint cavity.

The incision may be continued proximally through the sartorius and vastus medialis muscles in order to expose a supracondylar fracture.

CLOSURE:

The joint capsule and medial fascia are closed in one layer with nonabsorbable suture material. A Lembert pattern is used to prevent any suture material from penetrating the synovial membrane of the joint capsule.

COMMENTS:

For arthrotomy alone, medial exposure is used in preference to the lateral approach whenever possible. Cicatrix formation is hidden and the interior of the joint is more widely exposed with a medial incision.

Page 108

PLATE 46. APPROACH TO THE DISTAL END OF THE FEMUR AND THE STIFLE JOINT THROUGH A MEDIAL INCISION

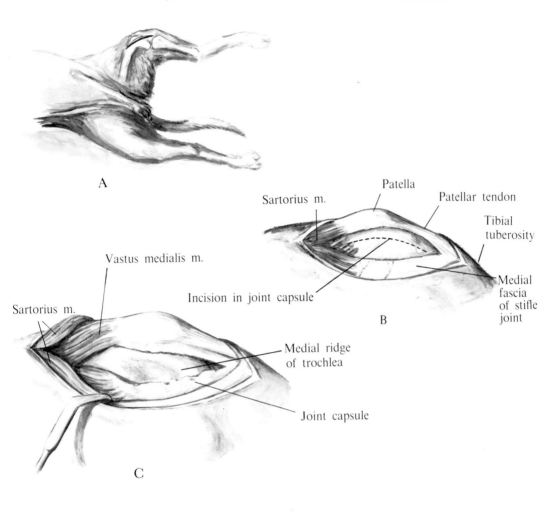

A

Sartorius m.

Patella

Patellar tendon

Tibial tuberosity

Incision in joint capsule

Medial fascia of stifle joint

B

Vastus medialis m.

Sartorius m.

Medial ridge of trochlea

Joint capsule

C

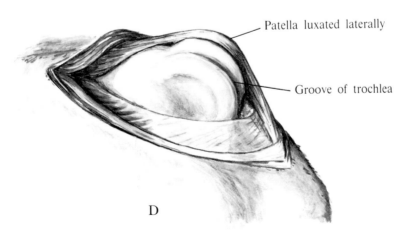

Patella luxated laterally

Groove of trochlea

D

Page 109

APPROACH TO THE DISTAL END OF THE FEMUR AND THE STIFLE JOINT WITH BILATERAL EXPOSURE

INDICATIONS:

1. Open reduction of comminuted supracondylar, intracondylar, and distal epiphyseal fractures of the femur.
2. Double Rush pin nailing of the femur.

EXPLANATORY NOTE:

Except for the skin incision, this procedure is a combination of the medial and lateral approaches to the distal end of the femur and the stifle joint (see Plates 45 and 46, pp. 107 and 109).

DESCRIPTION OF PROCEDURE:

A.   The double curved skin incision begins at the distal fourth of the femur and runs over the lateral trochlear ridge parallel to the patella. At the level of the middle of the patellar tendon, the incision turns to cross the tendon at a 45 degree angle and ends on the medial surface of the tibial tuberosity. The subcutaneous fascia is incised in the same manner. The medial skin flap and fascia are undermined and retracted medially.

B.   To expose the medial side, see illustrations B, C, and D of Plate 46.

C.   Entrance to the lateral side is shown in illustrations B, C, and D of Plate 45.

D.   The entire trochlear portion of the femur and the cranial compartment of the stifle joint are now exposed.

CLOSURE:

Suturing is done as previously explained for the medial and lateral approaches.

COMMENTS:

This approach may be combined with the Approach to the Shaft of the Femur (Plate 44, p. 105) to allow double Rush pin nailing of fractures in the lower end of the femur. The joint capsule need not be incised to insert these pins through the flat trochlear surfaces. This skin incision is the same as that made when Paatsama's technique for repair of a ruptured cranial cruciate ligament is performed. The incision is merely lengthened proximally to the level of the greater trochanter to allow the collection of a strip of fascia lata of suitable length.

PLATE 47. APPROACH TO THE DISTAL SHAFT OF THE FEMUR AND THE STIFLE JOINT WITH BILATERAL EXPOSURE

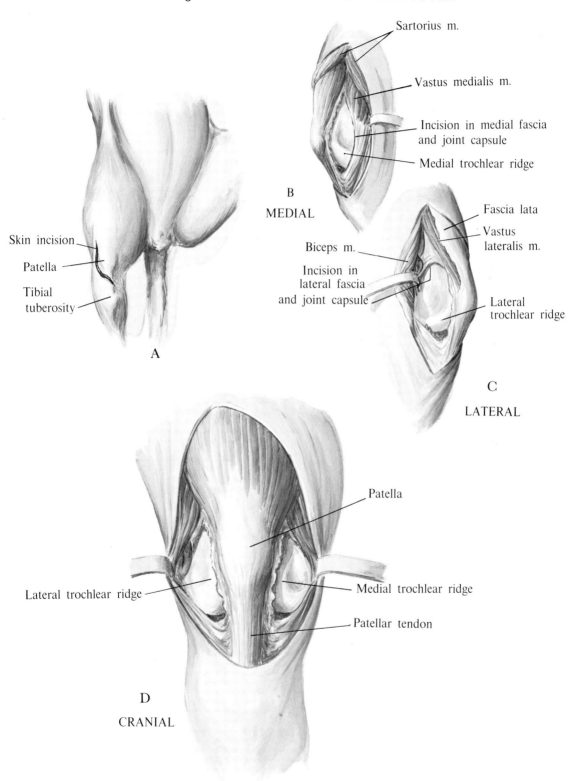

Sartorius m.

Vastus medialis m.

Incision in medial fascia and joint capsule

Medial trochlear ridge

B
MEDIAL

Fascia lata

Vastus lateralis m.

Biceps m.

Incision in lateral fascia and joint capsule

Lateral trochlear ridge

C
LATERAL

Skin incision

Patella

Tibial tuberosity

A

Patella

Lateral trochlear ridge

Medial trochlear ridge

Patellar tendon

D
CRANIAL

Page 111

APPROACH TO THE STIFLE JOINT THROUGH A MEDIAL TRANSVERSE INCISION

INDICATIONS:

1. Removal of the medial meniscus.
2. Removal of loose bodies from the caudal compartment of the joint.
3. Repair of the medial collateral ligament.

DESCRIPTION OF PROCEDURE:

A. The patella and the distal border of the medial femoral condyle are the landmarks for the incision, which starts medial to the patella and angles distally and caudally over the edge of the condyle.

B. The subcutaneous fascia is incised in the same line. The skin margins are mobilized and retracted so as to expose the medial fascia of the stifle joint. The medial fascia and joint capsule are incised from the lower edge of the patella to the medial collateral ligament. Do not incise the ligament. A branch of the medial genicular artery must be ligated as it crosses the incision.

C. By retraction of the caudal belly of the sartorius muscle, the joint incision can be lengthened into the caudal compartment of the joint if care is taken to avoid the medial collateral ligament.

CLOSURE:

The joint capsule and the medial fascia are closed in one layer by using a Lembert pattern if nonabsorbable suture material is used. The use of this pattern will prevent any suture material from being placed inside the joint.

PLATE 48. APPROACH TO THE STIFLE JOINT THROUGH A MEDIAL TRANSVERSE INCISION

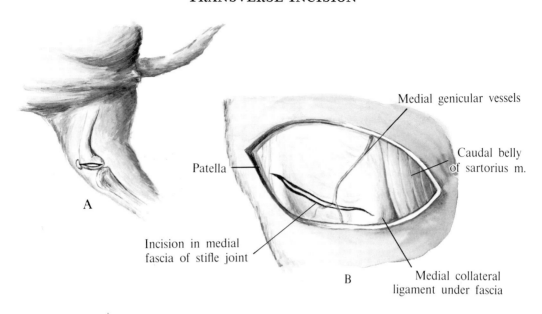

A

Medial genicular vessels

Caudal belly of sartorius m.

Patella

Incision in medial fascia of stifle joint

Medial collateral ligament under fascia

B

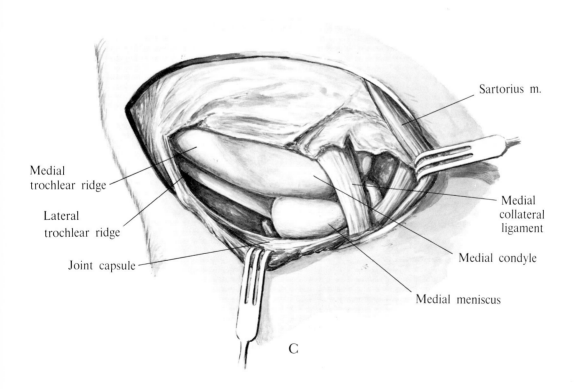

Sartorius m.

Medial trochlear ridge

Lateral trochlear ridge

Joint capsule

Medial collateral ligament

Medial condyle

Medial meniscus

C

Page 113

APPROACH TO THE PATELLA

INDICATION:

Patellectomy.

DESCRIPTION OF PROCEDURE:

A. A straight skin incision is made medial to the cranial midline of the limb. The length of the incision is approximately three times that of the patella. The subcutaneous fascia is incised on the same line and is undermined on the lateral side to expose the patellar and quadriceps tendons.

B. The skin is retracted and the stifle joint strongly flexed to fix the patella. A midline incision commences in the tendon of the quadriceps, continues through the periosteum of the patella, and ends in the patellar tendon.

C. The scalpel blade is used to elevate the periosteum from the patella by working from each end toward the center of the bone. Since the fibers of the quadriceps and patellar tendons attach to this periosteum, every effort is made to elevate the periosteal layer intact and thus to preserve continuity between the two tendons.

D. Periosteal elevation continues to the joint capsule, which is then incised to free the patella. The towel clamp is a convenient tool for grasping the patella.

CLOSURE:

The defect left by the removal of the patella is closed longitudinally. Nonabsorbable material is used, and the sutures are placed so as not to penetrate the joint capsule.

PLATE 49. APPROACH TO THE PATELLA

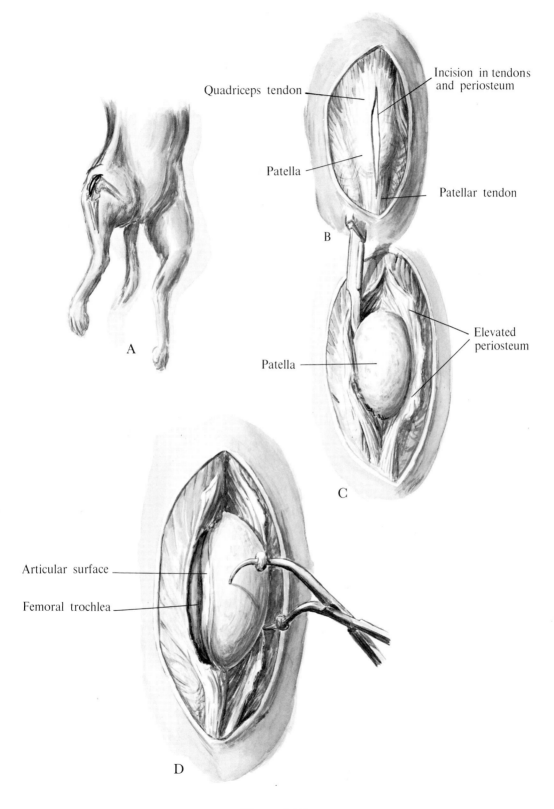

Quadriceps tendon

Incision in tendons and periosteum

Patella

Patellar tendon

B

A

Elevated periosteum

Patella

C

Articular surface

Femoral trochlea

D

APPROACH TO THE SHAFT OF THE TIBIA

INDICATION:

Open reduction of fractures in any area of the shaft.

DESCRIPTION OF PROCEDURE:

A. The skin incision is made directly over the medial aspect of the bone. The subcutaneous fascia is opened in the same line as the skin incision, care being taken to protect the dorsal branch of the saphenous vessels and nerve crossing the field at the midshaft. The saphenous vessels and nerve are freed and retracted in the appropriate direction – either proximally or distally depending on the area of the bone it is necessary to expose.

B. The bone is exposed by incising the deep crural fascia on the medial shaft of the bone. The cranial tibial, popliteus, and long digital flexor muscles may be reflected from the bone by subperiosteal elevation if necessary.

CLOSURE:

The deep crural fascia must be closed by sutures in order to preserve the insertion of the sartorius, gracilis, and semitendinosus muscles on the tibia.

Page 116

PLATE 50. APPROACH TO THE SHAFT OF THE TIBIA

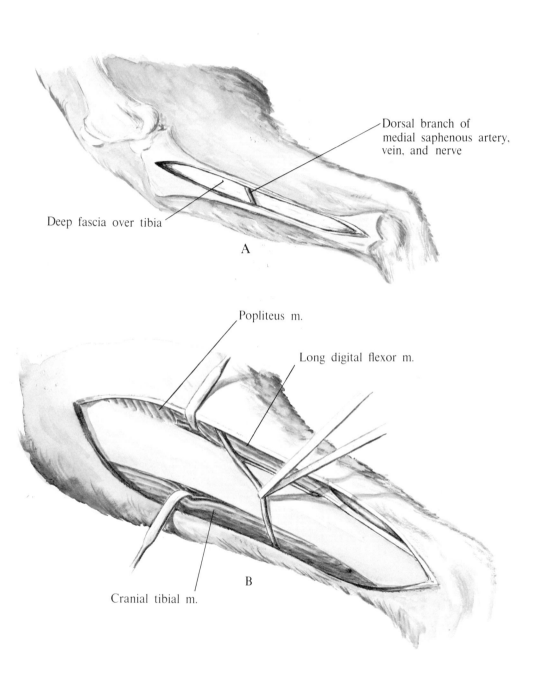

Dorsal branch of
medial saphenous artery,
vein, and nerve

Deep fascia over tibia

A

Popliteus m.

Long digital flexor m.

Cranial tibial m.

B

APPROACH TO THE DISTAL END OF THE TIBIA AND THE HOCK JOINT THROUGH A MEDIAL INCISION

INDICATION:

Open reduction of fractures of the medial malleolus of the tibia.

DESCRIPTION OF PROCEDURE:

A. The skin incision is started on the medial surface of the distal end of the tibia and continued across the joint to end at the middle of the tarsal area.

B. The subcutaneous fascia is incised on the same line, undermined, and retracted with the skin.

An incision is next made through the deep fascia and periosteum, commencing cranial and proximal to the prominence of the malleolus and continuing distally parallel to the tibial collateral ligament. The distal half of this incision will enter the joint capsule.

C. Subperiosteal elevation will allow the freeing of the dense fascia overlying the bone sufficiently to expose a limited area of the medial malleolus. The origin of the tibial collateral ligament on the malleolus should not be totally disrupted.

CLOSURE:

Interrupted sutures are used to close the incision in the deep fascia. No special attempt is made to close the synovial portion of the joint capsule.

PLATE 51. APPROACH TO THE DISTAL END OF THE TIBIA AND THE HOCK JOINT THROUGH A MEDIAL INCISION

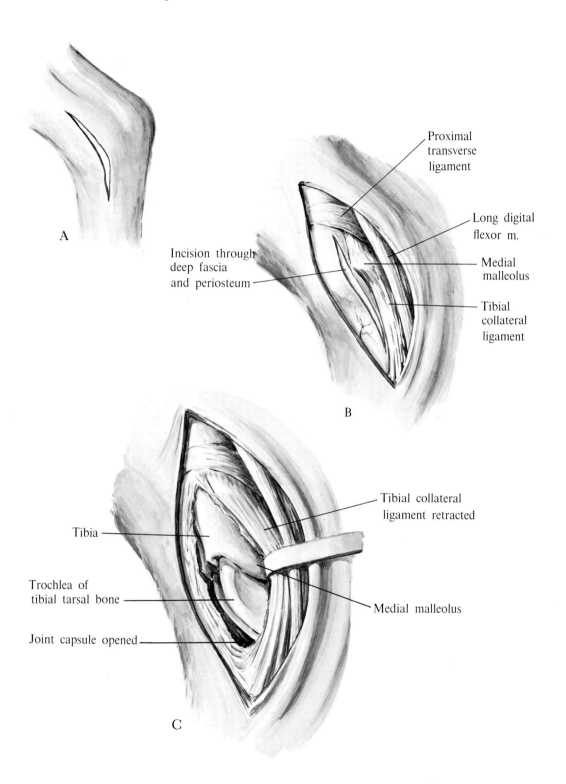

A

Incision through
deep fascia
and periosteum

Proximal
transverse
ligament

Long digital
flexor m.

Medial
malleolus

Tibial
collateral
ligament

B

Tibia

Trochlea of
tibial tarsal bone

Joint capsule opened

Tibial collateral
ligament retracted

Medial malleolus

C

APPROACH TO THE DISTAL END OF THE TIBIA AND FIBULA AND THE HOCK JOINT THROUGH A LATERAL INCISION

INDICATIONS:

1. Open reduction of fractures of the lateral malleolus of the fibula.
2. Open reduction of supramalleolar fractures of the tibia.
3. Open reduction of luxations of the hock joint.

DESCRIPTION OF PROCEDURE:

A. A curved skin incision is made over the lateral surface of the joint, commencing proximally at the level of the lateral saphenous vein and continuing distally to the level of the intertarsal joint.

B. The subcutaneous fascia is incised on the same line as the skin and is retracted with the skin. All the deep structures are covered by dense fascial tissue and are poorly visualized at this point.

The deep fascial band overlying the distal end of the bones is incised parallel to the cranial border of the fibularis longus tendon, care being taken to avoid cutting the tendon.

C. The caudal part of the fascial band must be elevated subperiosteally to expose the entire lateral malleolus. If the joint is to be opened, the joint capsule is incised parallel to the distal end of the bones.

CLOSURE:

The carpal band is rejoined by one mattress suture. The joint capsule is not closed, but the subcutaneous fascia is sutured carefully in order to completely cover the joint.

PLATE 52. APPROACH TO THE DISTAL END OF THE TIBIA AND FIBULA AND THE HOCK JOINT THROUGH A LATERAL INCISION

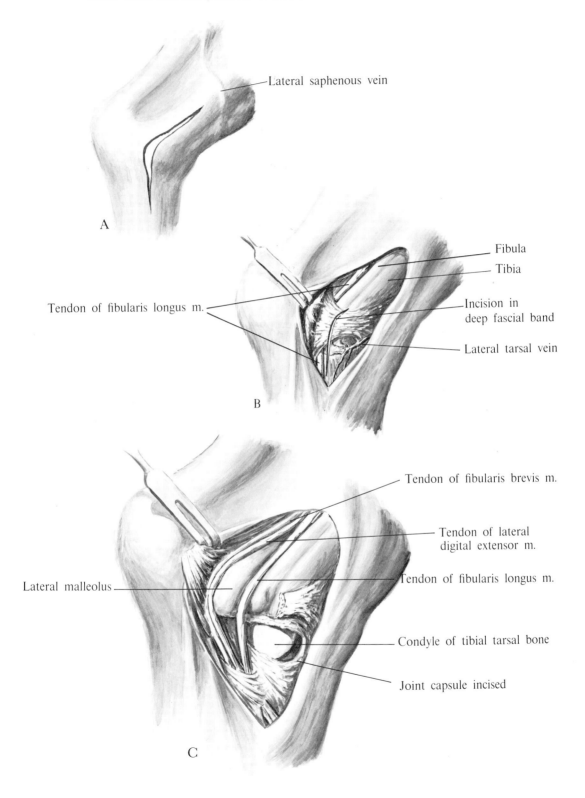

Lateral saphenous vein

A

Fibula

Tibia

Tendon of fibularis longus m.

Incision in deep fascial band

Lateral tarsal vein

B

Tendon of fibularis brevis m.

Tendon of lateral digital extensor m.

Tendon of fibularis longus m.

Lateral malleolus

Condyle of tibial tarsal bone

Joint capsule incised

C

Page 121

APPROACH TO THE TUBER CALCANEI OF THE FIBULAR TARSAL BONE

INDICATION:

Open reduction of fractures of the bone.

DESCRIPTION OF PROCEDURE:

A. The skin incision is straight and extends the length of the caudolateral surface of the fibular tarsal bone.

B. The subcutaneous fascia is incised similarly and is retracted with the skin following its undermining and elevation from the deep fascia. The tendon of the abductor digiti quinti muscle and an underlying tendon of the superficial digital flexor muscle should now be visible on the caudolateral border of the bone. An incision is made through the deep fascia and periosteum just cranial to these structures.

C. Elevation and reflection of the periosteum will allow retraction of the abductor digiti quinti tendon sufficiently to expose the lateral surface of the bone.

CLOSURE:

One row of interrupted sutures is placed in the deep fascia and periosteum.

PLATE 53. APPROACH TO THE TUBER CALCANEI OF THE FIBULAR TARSAL BONE

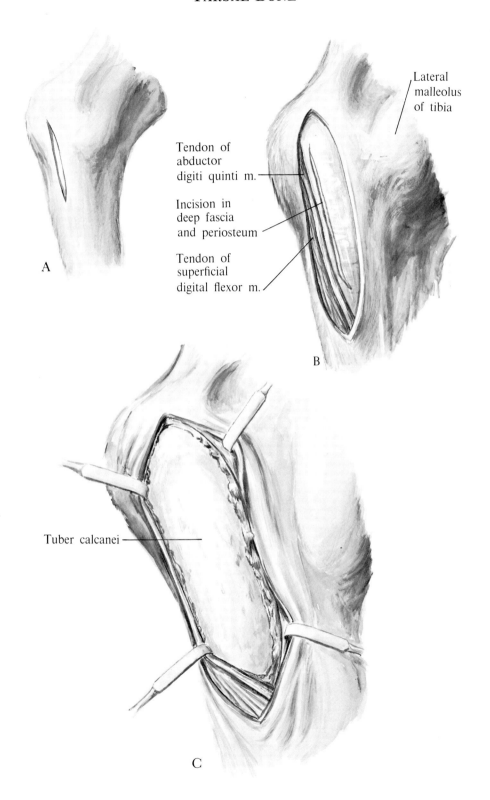

A

Lateral malleolus of tibia

Tendon of abductor digiti quinti m.

Incision in deep fascia and periosteum

Tendon of superficial digital flexor m.

B

Tuber calcanei

C

APPROACH TO THE CENTRAL TARSAL BONE

INDICATIONS:

1. Open reduction of fractures of the bone.
2. Excision of necrotic fragments of bone and their replacement with prosthesis.

DESCRIPTION OF PROCEDURE:

A. A vertical incision approximately 2 inches long is made just medial to the saphenous vein and is centered over the tarsal region.

B. The subcutaneous fascia and skin are undermined and retracted. The deep fascia is incised between the tendon of the cranial tibial muscle and the branching vessel from the saphenous vein.

C. Vigorous undermining is required to elevate and retract the deep fascia from the surface of the central tarsal bone.

CLOSURE:

The deep fascia is joined by one row of interrupted sutures.

COMMENTS:

Fractures of this bone occur almost exclusively in track-raced greyhounds, and always in the right, or outside, foot.

PLATE 54. APPROACH TO THE CENTRAL TARSAL BONE

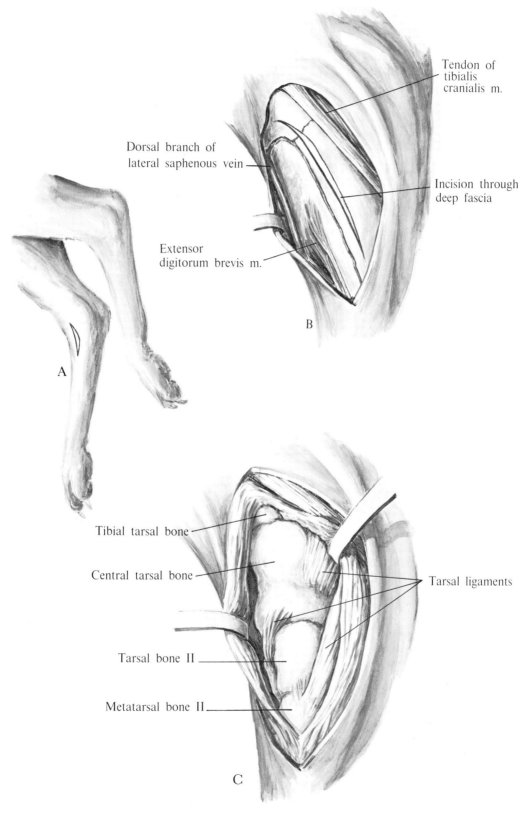

Tendon of
tibialis
cranialis m.

Dorsal branch of
lateral saphenous vein

Incision through
deep fascia

Extensor
digitorum brevis m.

B

A

Tibial tarsal bone

Central tarsal bone

Tarsal ligaments

Tarsal bone II

Metatarsal bone II

C

APPROACHES TO THE METATARSAL BONES

INDICATION:

Open reduction of fractures.

DESCRIPTION OF PROCEDURE:

The anatomy shown here is considerably simplified compared to that in the live animal. Only important structures are shown; other elements such as small tendons and blood vessels have been omitted. In an average sized dog these structures are so small as to preclude their identification and preservation during surgery.

The incisional technique varies according to the bone or bones to be exposed. A single bone is approached by an incision directly over the bone, and two adjoining bones by an incision between them. If more than two bones need be exposed, two parallel longitudinal incisions or a single curved incision can be used. The curved incision commences at the proximal end of metatarsal II, runs laterally to the midshaft of metatarsal V, and then curves medially again to end over the distal end of metatarsal II. The crescent-shaped skin flap can be elevated and retracted to expose a large part of all four bones.

Metatarsals II and V can be approached directly, without elevation of any important tendons or vessels. The deep fascia is incised and elevated to allow visualization of these bones. Exposure of metatarsal bones III and IV requires the undermining and retraction of the tendon of the long digital extensor muscle and the accompanying blood vessels.

CLOSURE:

Deep fascia is closed to insure that tendons and vessels are securely held in their proper positions.

COMMENTS:

A deep layer of small blood vessels is found on and between the bones. These vessels are too small to avoid in most animals and the resulting hemorrhage must be controlled by tamponade. The use of a tourniquet is very helpful when the operative site is in the regions below the hock or radiocarpal joint. Do not leave the tourniquet in place for more than one hour, and apply a snug bandage for 72 hours postoperatively to control oozing hemorrhage at the operative site.

PLATE 55. APPROACHES TO THE METATARSAL BONES

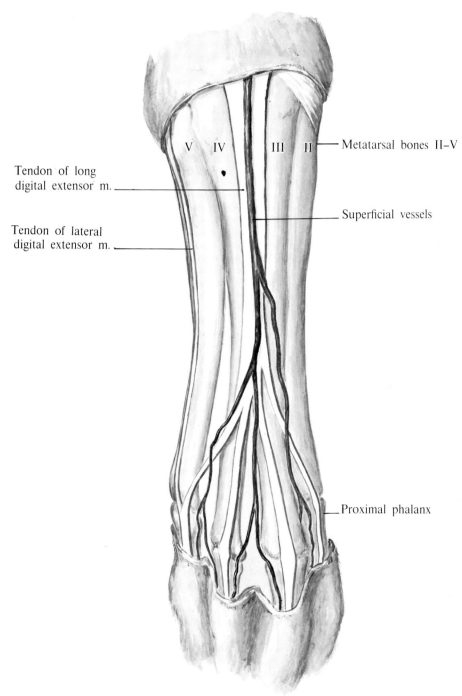

V IV III II — Metatarsal bones II–V

Tendon of long
digital extensor m.

Superficial vessels

Tendon of lateral
digital extensor m.

Proximal phalanx

Dorsal aspect of right metatarsus with skin removed

INDEX

Page 130

Page 131